SAMANTHA PETEREIN

The Lunar Herbalist

Harnessing Moon Phases for Growth & Healing

This book was professionally typeset on Reedsy.
Find out more at reedsy.com

To all the souls who are walking the path to healing:
May you find peace in knowing you are never alone.

Contents

A Word on Herbs and Safety

While the information in this book is grounded in tradition and personal practice, it is important to remember that herbs can affect people in different ways. The guidance offered here is for informational purposes only, and it's always best to consult with a healthcare provider before incorporating new herbs into your wellness routine, especially if you are pregnant, nursing, or have existing health conditions.

Prologue

There's a rhythm to everything. The moon, the tides, the seasons, even our breath—all flow in cycles, a dance of expansion and release, light and shadow. For as long as I can remember, I've felt the quiet pull of these cycles, even when life seemed anything but steady.

I've spent much of my life trying to keep everything together, caring for others, pushing through challenges, and silencing my own needs. But when my health took a sudden turn, forcing me to face a diagnosis I wasn't prepared for, the threads I'd been holding onto so tightly began to unravel. My world felt heavy, uncertain, and out of my control. The anxiety, the fear, the darkness—it all seemed too much to carry.

That's when I found myself turning to the moon.

I started observing its cycles—its gentle rise and fall in the sky, its moments of fullness and its quiet retreats into shadow. I began to realize that the moon mirrored my own internal landscape. There were days when I felt vibrant, full of light, and others when I needed to retreat, to heal, to let go. The moon, with its unchanging rhythm, reminded me that no matter where I was in my own cycle—whether in the brightness of growth or the shadow of release—it was all part of a larger journey.

Nature, too, became my refuge. The simple act of brewing an herbal tea, tending to the plants in my garden, or walking barefoot on the earth became grounding practices that soothed the chaos inside me. I found that when I aligned myself with the natural rhythms of the moon and the healing power of herbs, I could tap into a deeper sense of balance and peace, even in the midst of life's storms.

This book is an offering—a way to share the tools, practices, and wisdom that have guided me through my own healing. It's a reminder that healing is not linear. Like the phases of the moon, we ebb and flow, and that's okay. Each phase has its purpose, and every moment of light and shadow contributes to our growth.

As you read these pages, I invite you to slow down, to listen to the whispers of nature, and to honor the cycles that shape your life. This is your journey, your sacred dance with the moon and the earth, and there is beauty in every phase.

May you find peace, healing, and connection as you embrace your own rhythm.

Welcome to the journey.

– Samantha Peterein

1

Exploring the Magick of the Moon and Herbs

For as long as humanity has existed, we've looked to the moon as a source of wonder, power, and guidance. Its phases have shaped not only the tides but also the rhythms of our lives, from planting cycles to spiritual practices. In this chapter, we will dive deep into the magick of the moon, exploring how its phases influence our emotions, energy, and personal growth. By understanding this, we can enhance our connection to the natural world and our well-being.

Throughout history, the moon has been revered as a cosmic force that mirrors the ebb and flow of life. Many ancient cultures—from the Egyptians to the Celts—recognized the moon's influence on both nature and human emotion. In modern times, while we may understand the scientific basis for the moon's pull on the tides, the emotional and energetic impact of the lunar cycle on our bodies and minds still resonates deeply with those who seek to align with its rhythm.

The Interconnection of Moon Phases and Human Energy

The moon affects not just the physical world but also our internal landscapes. Just as the gravitational pull of the moon influences the tides, it is believed to influence the emotional tides within us. Each phase of the moon carries a distinct energy that can be harnessed for healing, growth, and transformation. By working with the moon's cycles, we can synchronize our personal intentions with nature's natural flow, enhancing our ability to manifest and release what no longer serves us.

Lunar Energy and the Human Body

Ancient civilizations were incredibly attuned to the cycles of the moon and recognized that the moon's phases aligned with physical and emotional rhythms. In Traditional Chinese Medicine (TCM), for instance, practitioners use lunar cycles to understand the balance of yin (passive, receptive energy) and yang (active, outward energy). The New Moon, a time of stillness, is a deeply yin phase, ideal for introspection and setting new intentions. The Full Moon, on the other hand, is yang, representing fullness, celebration, and culmination.

Our bodies, being made up of 60% water, are naturally affected by the moon's gravitational pull, just like the tides. Studies suggest that the moon's influence can affect sleep patterns, moods, and even fertility. By tuning in to how we feel during each phase, we can work with our body's natural rhythm rather than against it, allowing for greater flow in our daily lives.

Aligning with the Moon for Healing

Healing with the moon is about more than just rituals; it's about developing a relationship with the cycles of nature and aligning our personal healing journeys with them. In times of emotional or physical imbalance, working with specific moon phases can help guide us back to a place of inner peace.

For example, during the New Moon, when the energy is reflective and quiet, we can turn inward and set intentions for our personal growth. This is a perfect time for creating new herbal remedies, setting long-term wellness goals, or beginning practices like journaling or meditation to help solidify our path.

As the moon waxes and the energy builds, we can take action toward those goals. The waxing phase is a powerful time for planting seeds—both figuratively and literally—allowing us to invest in our physical and emotional wellness. Herbal crafting during this phase is ideal for creating remedies that promote growth, such as tonics for vitality or energizing teas.

The Full Moon, which is associated with the height of emotional and spiritual power, offers a perfect opportunity for releasing old wounds, limiting beliefs, or toxic behaviors. During this phase, healing rituals that incorporate herbs like sage or lavender are ideal for emotional release, helping to clear away what no longer serves us and create space for new growth.

Finally, the waning moon brings the energy of release, where we can focus on letting go of the physical and emotional clutter in our lives. This phase encourages us to rest, restore, and integrate the lessons we've learned, preparing us for the next cycle of healing.

Herbs and the Moon: A Symbiotic Relationship

Just as the moon affects the ocean's tides, many believe it also influences the potency of herbs and their healing properties. Traditional herbalists have long followed the lunar cycles when planting, harvesting, and crafting remedies, believing that the moon's energy enhances the qualities of plants.

During the New Moon, herbs associated with new beginnings and fresh energy—such as rosemary, peppermint, or basil—are often harvested to capture the lunar energy of growth and intention.

As the moon waxes, the energy builds, and herbs like ginger, ginseng, or nettle—known for their energizing and vitalizing properties—are said to be most potent during this time.

At the Full Moon, herbs that support emotional balance and reflection, such as lavender, chamomile, and rose, are harvested and used in rituals to release negative energy and calm the mind.

Finally, during the Waning Moon, herbs associated with release and cleansing, such as sage, lemongrass, and thyme, are ideal for rituals focused on letting go and clearing space.

My Personal Journey with the Moon and Herbs

The moon has been a constant presence in my healing journey. For years, I battled anxiety, burnout, and emotional imbalance, feeling disconnected from myself and the natural world around me. It wasn't until I began exploring the cycles of the moon that I found a framework that grounded me and helped me make sense of my healing process. Aligning my wellness practices with the lunar phases gave me a sense of purpose, reminding me that healing, like the moon's phases, is a cyclical and ongoing process.

As I deepened my practice, I found ways to incorporate the moon's energy into my use of herbs. Whether it was preparing a tea blend or setting intentions, these small rituals helped me stay connected to my goals, fostering balance and clarity in my life. Each phase of the moon offered its own lessons, and by aligning my herbal practices accordingly, I felt more in tune with the natural cycles of growth and release.

My practice has grown beyond personal healing—I now see it as part of my calling to serve and support the collective. I've come to believe that by sharing these practices, I can help others tap into their own innate wisdom and healing potential. Just as the moon reflects the cycles of nature, it also reflects the cycles within ourselves. It is my hope that through these pages, you will find the tools to connect with those cycles and bring greater balance into your life.

What You Will Learn in This Book

In this book, you'll discover how to work with the moon's phases to enhance your own wellness practices, how to use herbs at the right times for their most potent effects, and how to create personal rituals that will support your healing journey.

Each chapter is designed to guide you through the different phases of the moon, offering herbal remedies, rituals, and reflections to help you align with the lunar cycle. You'll learn:

- How to harness the energy of each moon phase to support personal growth, manifestation, and healing.

- The best herbs to use for each phase of the lunar cycle, and how to craft your own teas, tinctures, and salves.
- Practical rituals and meditations that will help you connect with the energy of the moon and enhance your spiritual and physical well-being.

2

The History and Magick of Lunar Healing

Since the dawn of humanity, the moon has been a guiding light, both physically and spiritually. Ancient peoples used the moon to mark time, navigate, and structure their rituals and ceremonies. These civilizations believed that the cycles of the moon reflected the cycles of life itself—birth, growth, death, and rebirth. The moon was regarded as both a cosmic clock and a powerful spiritual force. The reverence each culture showed toward the moon is mirrored in their unique rituals and celebrations.

Mesopotamia: The Birthplace of Lunar Calendars

In the cradle of civilization, ancient Mesopotamians were among the first to record and study the cycles of the moon. They recognized its connection to the rhythms of the Earth, from the tides to agricultural seasons. The Mesopotamians worshipped the moon god Sin (Nanna), who they believed controlled time and fate. Farmers timed their planting and harvesting to the phases of the moon, believing that its energy directly influenced the success of their crops. The moon was seen as a benevolent force that could guide them toward abundance and prosperity.

In addition to its influence on agriculture, Mesopotamians used the moon as a spiritual compass. Their priests observed the phases of the moon to predict celestial events, such as eclipses, which they believed were omens sent by the gods. Rituals and offerings to Sin were performed during specific lunar phases, aligning their religious practices with the cosmos.

Egypt: Lunar Goddesses and the Cycle of Life

In ancient Egypt, the moon was personified as both the god Thoth and the goddess Isis, each representing the moon's dual influence over life and death. Isis, in particular, was associated with healing, fertility, and renewal. Egyptian healers would craft herbal remedies and perform rituals during specific moon phases, believing that the energy of the lunar cycle would enhance their effectiveness. The ancient Egyptians also used a lunar calendar to structure their agricultural and religious festivals, aligning their lives with the moon's cycles for optimal growth and spiritual connection.

One of the most significant lunar rituals in ancient Egypt was the "Feast of Osiris," which was held under the light of the Full Moon. This festival symbolized renewal and resurrection, and it was believed that the Full Moon's energy helped guide the spirit of Osiris through the underworld, ensuring the fertility of the land. Healers during this time would craft herbal balms and oils infused with moonlit herbs, using these to anoint the body and promote both physical and spiritual healing.

Greece and Rome: The Lunar Goddess and Healing

In ancient Greece, the moon was represented by the goddess Selene, who drove her chariot across the night sky, illuminating the darkness. Selene was revered for her beauty and power, symbolizing clarity, reflection, and emotional healing. Greek healers would often conduct their rituals under the Full Moon, believing that its light could amplify the potency of their herbs and spiritual work. The Roman counterpart to Selene, Luna, carried similar symbolism, representing the feminine force of intuition, emotional depth, and nurturing energy.

One particular festival, the Roman "Lemuria," was held during the dark, waning moon, and was centered on purging negative spirits from households. During this festival, families would prepare bundles of protective herbs, such as sage and rosemary, which were hung in doorways to clear negative energy and ward off unwanted spirits. The association of the Waning Moon with protection and banishing continues to influence modern lunar magick practices.

Both civilizations believed that by working with the moon's cycles, they could harness its energy to enhance healing, personal growth, and transformation. This connection to the moon and its phases laid the groundwork for the practices of lunar magick and herbal healing that continue to this day.

Modern Adaptations of Lunar Healing Practices

In recent years, there has been a growing resurgence of interest in lunar magick and holistic healing practices. Many modern healers and spiritual practitioners are rediscovering the power of working with the moon's phases, integrating ancient wisdom with contemporary wellness practices. For those living busy, modern lives, adapting lunar practices can feel daunting. However, with small, intentional steps, these ancient rituals can easily be adapted to suit the demands of contemporary life without losing their depth or magickal potency.

New Moon: Setting Intentions in the Digital Age

In today's world, where our daily schedules are often packed with commitments, many people feel disconnected from nature. One of the simplest ways to reconnect with the energy of the New Moon is through intentional journaling. Even a few minutes of writing down your personal goals or reflections on what you wish to invite into your life can help you align with the New Moon's energy of beginnings.

For those who feel disconnected from their creative side, consider using a digital moon phase tracker or app to remind you when it's time to set your intentions. You could also create a vision board on your phone or tablet, using images that inspire the goals you are working toward. Technology can be a tool for lunar magick, allowing us to weave ancient practices into the fabric of modern life.

Waxing Moon: Building Energy and Momentum

During the Waxing Moon, when the energy of growth is at its peak, consider incorporating simple, everyday rituals that help you build momentum. Instead of feeling the need to perform elaborate ceremonies, find small ways to focus on growth—whether it's tending to houseplants, creating a nourishing herbal tea blend, or organizing your workspace. These acts of care and attention align with the Waxing Moon's energy of expansion.

For those short on time, creating a Waxing Moon playlist with songs that motivate and energize you can be a quick way to channel this lunar energy. Play this music while you prepare your meals, exercise, or commute to work to infuse your day with the energy of growth.

Full Moon: Reflecting and Releasing with Modern Tools

The Full Moon is traditionally a time for reflection and release. One of the simplest ways to practice this in modern life is through meditation or a mindful walk outdoors. However, for those who struggle with time constraints, a modern twist on this practice is to use apps like Calm or Insight Timer to guide you through a 10- to 15-minute Full Moon meditation.

Additionally, consider creating a digital "release" ceremony by writing down things you wish to let go of and deleting them from your device after the Full Moon. This symbolic act of letting go can be just as powerful as burning physical papers, especially when combined with breathwork or a short candlelight ceremony.

Waning Moon: Rest and Reset for Busy Lives

The Waning Moon is all about release, renewal, and rest. In today's fast-paced world, many people struggle to slow down. Use the energy of the Waning Moon as a reminder to schedule intentional breaks in your day, even if they are just five minutes long. Focus on releasing tension from your body through quick stretching exercises, or clear mental clutter by practicing deep breathing.

If you're interested in working with herbs during the Waning Moon, you can make a simple herbal cleansing spray with ingredients like sage, rosemary, and peppermint essential oils. This can be spritzed around your home or workspace to refresh the energy and create a sense of calm and renewal without needing to conduct a full cleansing ritual.

Adapting Lunar Rituals for Modern Spaces

You don't need access to a grand outdoor space or uninterrupted hours of time to practice lunar magick. Modern lunar practitioners often live in apartments, cities, or other places where outdoor rituals may not be feasible. Consider crafting a small "moon altar" in your home, a dedicated space where you can connect with lunar energy. This could be as simple as a windowsill with a candle, a crystal, and a journal.

For those who travel frequently or have limited space, consider creating a portable lunar ritual kit. This could include a small vial of moon-charged water, a sprig of rosemary, and a roll-on essential oil blend corresponding to the current moon phase. With these small tools, you can bring the magick of the moon into any environment, allowing for continued alignment with its cycles even on the go.

3

The New Moon: Beginnings, Intentions, and Manifestation

The New Moon is a time of quiet potential—a blank slate in the lunar cycle where everything is possible, but nothing has yet taken form. When the moon is in its darkest phase, it invites us to turn inward, reflect, and set intentions for what we wish to manifest in our lives. This phase is ideal for fresh starts, new beginnings, and planting seeds of intention for future growth. In this chapter, we will explore how the energy of the New Moon can support your personal and spiritual journey, how to align with this phase using herbs, and how to craft rituals that harness its magick.

The Energy of the New Moon: A Time for Renewal

Though often unseen in the night sky, the New Moon's influence is powerful and transformative. This phase represents the start of a new lunar cycle, offering us the opportunity to begin again. Energetically, the New Moon is a time of introspection and self-reflection, encouraging us to pause, turn inward, and assess where we are on our personal journey. What are we carrying that no longer serves us? What dreams or goals do we wish to manifest moving forward?

In many ancient cultures, the New Moon was seen as a sacred time for setting intentions and making commitments. Communities would gather in ceremony to offer their prayers, plant crops, or make vows aligned with the energy of renewal. Just as seeds are planted in the earth, our intentions are planted in our subconscious during this time, ready to grow as the moon waxes and its energy builds.

From a spiritual perspective, the New Moon invites us to honor both endings and beginnings. It is a powerful time to release what is no longer needed and to set intentions for the future. By aligning with this energy, we open ourselves to new possibilities and opportunities for growth.

Setting Intentions with the New Moon

Intention-setting is one of the most powerful practices associated with the New Moon. This is a time to gain clarity about your desires, goals, and dreams. What do you want to bring into your life? What seeds do you want to plant for your future?

Setting intentions during the New Moon is not merely wishful thinking—it is a practice of mindfulness and focused energy. When you set an intention, you are actively aligning your thoughts, emotions, and actions with your desired outcome. This practice not only helps you stay focused on your goals but also creates a sense of accountability, allowing you to take practical steps toward manifesting your desires.

How to Set Intentions During the New Moon

1. Find a Quiet Space: Create a peaceful environment where you can be alone with your thoughts. Light a candle or some incense to create a sacred, calming space.
2. Reflect: Spend time reflecting on where you are in your life and what you want to change or manifest. What challenges are you currently facing? What are your deepest desires and aspirations?
3. Write Down Your Intentions: Grab a journal and write down your intentions for this lunar cycle. Be as specific as possible. For example, instead of saying, "I want to be healthier," you could write, "I intend to walk for 30 minutes every day and make nourishing choices for my body."
4. Visualize: Once you've written down your intentions, close your eyes and visualize them coming to life. See yourself already living in alignment with your intentions. Feel the emotions associated with achieving your goals.
5. Plant the Seed: Just as farmers plant seeds during the New Moon, consider your intentions as seeds you are planting in your subconscious. Trust that, just like seeds, your intentions will grow and manifest as the moon's energy builds.
6. Stay Open: Release attachment to the outcome and allow the universe to work in its own time. Trust that your intentions are already in motion.

Herbs Associated with the New Moon

The New Moon is a time for clarity, purification, and new beginnings, and the herbs associated with this phase reflect those qualities. These herbs help us cleanse and clear our energy, ground ourselves, and set a strong foundation for manifesting our intentions.

- Sage (Salvia officinalis): Traditionally used for cleansing and purification, sage is rooted in Indigenous North American spiritual practices (specifically smudging) and ancient Greek and Roman healing traditions. For this book, we focus on its general cleansing properties, often used to clear negative energy and create space for new beginnings. Be mindful of the cultural significance of sage, particularly in Indigenous communities, and approach its use with respect.
- Jasmine (Jasminum officinale): Known for its association with the moon and intuition, jasmine enhances spiritual awareness and clarity. Its calming scent is perfect for meditation and intention-setting rituals during the New Moon.
- Rosemary (Rosmarinus officinalis): Often linked to clarity and focus, rosemary sharpens the mind and enhances memory, making it an excellent herb for setting specific goals and staying committed to your intentions.
- Lemon Balm (Melissa officinalis): Known for its calming and soothing properties, lemon balm helps to reduce stress and anxiety, making it easier to reflect and focus on your true desires during the New Moon.

Herbal Ritual for New Moon Intention-Setting

To enhance your intention-setting practice, consider incorporating a simple herbal ritual using these New Moon herbs.

1. Create a Sacred Space: Begin by cleansing your space with burning sage or rosemary to clear away any stagnant energy.
2. Herbal Tea for Clarity: Brew a tea using jasmine, lemon balm, and a sprig

of rosemary. As you sip your tea, focus on your intentions for the coming lunar cycle. Allow the calming properties of the herbs to relax your mind and open you to receiving guidance.

3. Journal Your Intentions: After drinking your tea, write down your intentions in your journal. Be clear and specific, and feel the energy of each intention taking root in your subconscious.

4. Close the Ritual: End the ritual by expressing gratitude for the New Moon's energy and the herbs that supported your practice. Hold your hands over your heart and repeat the affirmation:

"I am open to new beginnings. I trust the universe to guide me toward my highest good."

Visualize your intentions manifesting as you say this affirmation.

Manifestation and Reflection Prompts for the New Moon

Use these prompts to guide your reflection and keep you focused on nurturing your intentions throughout the lunar cycle.

Manifestation Prompt:

- What seeds of intention are you ready to plant during this lunar cycle? Take a few minutes to sit quietly and reflect on your desires. Write down three specific goals or intentions that you want to focus on. Be clear and specific. Visualize yourself achieving these goals and think about the steps you can take during the Waxing Moon to help them grow.

Reflection Prompts:

- What steps am I actively taking to nurture the seeds of my intentions, and how can I ensure I stay on track?
- How do I approach challenges or obstacles that arise during the growth phase? What mindset will help me persevere?
- Where in my life am I seeing positive progress, and how can I build on that momentum?

Journaling Prompts:

- Reflect on your progress thus far. What are three actions you can take this week to move closer to your goals?
- Are there any areas where you've felt resistance or procrastination? Write down what's holding you back and how you can overcome it.
- What does the concept of growth mean to you, and how do you personally define success as you work toward your intentions?

Expanding Your New Moon Practice

The New Moon is an incredibly potent time for beginning new practices and integrating new approaches into your life. While intention-setting is a central part of this phase, there are other ways to deepen your connection to the New Moon's energy.

Here are some additional ways to expand your New Moon practice:

- Creative Visualization: Take time to meditate on the goals and desires you've set. Visualize them in great detail, imagining not only the outcome but also the steps you'll take to get there. Visualization can help solidify your intentions and align your subconscious mind with your conscious goals.

- Candle Magick: The New Moon's darkness is perfect for candle magick, where you can use the symbolism of lighting a candle to represent the start of something new. Choose a white or silver candle for purity and new beginnings, and as you light it, focus on your intentions growing with the increasing moonlight.

- Crystal Work: Work with crystals that resonate with new beginnings and manifestation. Stones such as moonstone (for new beginnings and intuition), labradorite (for transformation and creativity), or clear quartz (for amplifying energy) can be powerful tools during this phase. Place them on your altar or carry them with you as you work on your intentions.

- Herbal Baths: Prepare an herbal bath with New Moon herbs such as jasmine, lemon balm, and rosemary to cleanse your energy and prepare yourself for the new cycle ahead As you soak, focus on releasing any lingering doubts or fears, and open yourself up to new opportunities.

- Moon Water: Set out a jar of water under the New Moon to create "moon water." Although it's typically charged under the Full Moon, creating moon water during the New Moon can symbolize the planting of intentions. You can use this water in future rituals, add it to your bath, or even water your plants with it to infuse them with your intentions.

- Journaling for Clarity: Beyond setting intentions, journaling during the New Moon can help you uncover hidden desires, explore new ideas, and clarify what you truly want in your life. Allow your journaling practice to be an open exploration of the possibilities this lunar phase offers.

Closing Thoughts on the New Moon

The New Moon is a powerful time of potential and renewal, offering us the chance to reset, refocus, and plant the seeds of our intentions. It is a time for quiet introspection and mindful action, reminding us that every new beginning starts with a single step.

As you work with the energy of the New Moon, remember that manifestation is a process. The seeds you plant during this phase may take time to grow, but with patience, dedication, and trust in the natural cycles, they will flourish. This is not the phase for immediate results, but rather for creating a strong foundation on which to build your dreams.

The darkness of the New Moon invites us to look within, to find clarity and inspiration from our inner world. By aligning with this phase and committing to your personal growth, you will find that the New Moon provides you with the perfect opportunity to set yourself on the path toward your highest potential.

4

The Waxing Moon: Growth, Action, and Manifestation

As the moon moves from the New Moon into its waxing phases—first the Waxing Crescent, then the First Quarter, and finally the Waxing Gibbous—its light grows stronger and brighter. This increasing energy is mirrored in our own lives, making it a time for growth, forward movement, and action. During the Waxing Moon, the intentions set during the New Moon begin to take form, and we are encouraged to take deliberate steps toward manifesting our goals. In this chapter, we will explore the magick of the Waxing Moon, the herbs that align with this phase, and how to work with its powerful energy to bring your desires into reality.

The Energy of the Waxing Moon: Taking Action and Building Momentum

The Waxing Moon is a time of action and momentum. As the moon's light grows each night, it symbolizes the expansion of energy, focus, and potential in our own lives. This is the time to act on the intentions you set during the New Moon, nurturing the seeds of your desires and taking practical steps toward manifesting them.

While the New Moon is a time for introspection and planning, the Waxing Moon is all about movement and manifestation. It is the phase where you begin to build on the foundation you created, moving forward with confidence and determination. This is a time to cultivate discipline, commitment, and perseverance. Just as the moon gradually becomes more visible in the night sky, your goals become more tangible as you put in the work to make them a reality.

In many cultures, the Waxing Moon is associated with growth, abundance, and the building of personal power. It is a time when the universe supports forward motion, and the energy of expansion is all around us. Whether you are working on a personal project, a relationship, or your own inner growth, this is the phase where the energy of creation and manifestation is most potent.

How to Harness the Energy of the Waxing Moon

During the Waxing Moon, it is important to stay focused on your intentions and take actionable steps toward achieving your goals. This is not the time for passivity or hesitation. The energy of this phase supports clarity, action, and follow-through.

Tips for Harnessing Waxing Moon Energy:

1. Set Clear Goals: Revisit the intentions you set during the New Moon. Refine and clarify them if necessary. Write down specific, actionable goals that you can work toward during this phase.
2. Create a Plan of Action: Break your goals into smaller, manageable steps. What do you need to accomplish each day or week to move closer to your intention? Create a roadmap for yourself.
3. Stay Committed: The Waxing Moon is about persistence. Stay dedicated to your goals, even when challenges arise. This is the phase where your efforts will begin to bear fruit if you remain focused.
4. Use Affirmations: Positive affirmations can help keep you aligned with your intentions. Repeat affirmations that reinforce your confidence and determination, such as, "I am capable of achieving my goals," or "Every step I take brings me closer to my desires."
5. Take Action: Don't be afraid to take bold action during the Waxing Moon. This is the time to step out of your comfort zone, try new things, and take risks that align with your intentions.

Herbs Associated with the Waxing Moon

The Waxing Moon is a time for growth, energy, and action, and the herbs associated with this phase support these qualities. These herbs help us stay focused, energized, and motivated, while also providing balance to ensure that we don't burn out during this active phase.

- Rosemary (Rosmarinus officinalis): Known for its ability to enhance memory, clarity, and focus, rosemary is the perfect herb to work with during the Waxing Moon. Its invigorating scent sharpens the mind and helps keep you on track as you work toward your goals. Rosemary can be used in teas, baths, or burned as incense to clear mental fog and increase focus.

- Peppermint (Mentha piperita): Peppermint is a refreshing herb that supports mental clarity and focus. Its stimulating properties help clear away distractions, allowing you to stay focused on your goals. Peppermint can be used in teas, essential oils, or even added to your bath for a refreshing and energizing boost.
- Ginseng (Panax ginseng): Ginseng is a powerful adaptogen that supports stamina, resilience, and endurance. It is the perfect herb for those who need sustained energy to pursue their goals during the Waxing Moon. Ginseng can be taken as a tea or tincture to enhance vitality and focus.
- Ginger (Zingiber officinale): A powerful energizer, ginger is known for its ability to stimulate circulation and vitality. Whether consumed in tea or used in a bath, ginger can help boost your physical and mental energy during the Waxing Moon, making it easier to stay motivated and take action.

Herbal Ritual for the Waxing Moon: Energizing Tea for Growth

This herbal tea blend combines the energizing and focusing properties of rosemary, ginger, and peppermint to support you during the Waxing Moon. It will help you stay mentally sharp and physically energized as you work toward manifesting your intentions.

Ingredients:

- 1 tsp dried rosemary
- 1 tsp dried peppermint
- ½ tsp grated fresh ginger (or ¼ tsp dried ginger)

Instructions:

1. Boil a cup of water and add the herbs
2. Let the herbs steep for 10 minutes, allowing their energizing properties to infuse the water.
3. Strain the tea and sip it slowly, taking mindful breaths with each sip. Visualize the energy of the herbs entering your body, filling you with vitality and focus.
4. As you drink, repeat the affirmation: "I take inspired action toward manifesting my dreams." Allow this affirmation to anchor your intention and create a sense of momentum.
5. Once you've finished the tea, take a few moments to reflect on the steps you will take in the coming days to nurture your goals. Write them down in your journal to keep yourself accountable.

This simple tea ritual will help you align your energy with the Waxing Moon and stay focused on your path of growth and manifestation.

Manifestation and Reflection Prompts for the Waxing Moon

The Waxing Moon provides an ideal time to review your progress and realign your efforts toward manifestation. Reflect on the intentions you set during the New Moon and the steps you've taken so far.

Manifestation Prompt:

- Revisit the intentions you set during the New Moon. What steps have you taken so far to nurture your goals? Write down three specific actions you can take during the Waxing Moon to build momentum toward your desired outcome. Be as clear and specific as possible, and think about how you will stay accountable to these actions throughout the phase.

Reflection Prompts:

- What has come to fruition in my life since the New Moon? Reflect on what has already manifested or begun to take shape. How can you celebrate your achievements, no matter how big or small?
- What am I ready to release—emotionally, mentally, or physically—so that I can create space for new energy and experiences? Growth often requires letting go of what no longer serves us. This is the time to reflect on what might be holding you back and to release it in order to make room for new opportunities.
- How have I grown or evolved since setting my intentions, and what lessons have I learned during this cycle? Growth is not only about external achievements but also about internal shifts. Take a moment to reflect on any personal growth, insights, or lessons you've gained during this lunar cycle.

Journaling Prompts:

- Reflect on your journey from the New Moon to the Waxing Moon. Write down three things you are proud of accomplishing and any unexpected results that have arisen during this phase. How have your goals evolved since the beginning of the lunar cycle?
- What are you holding onto that no longer serves you? Consider any habits, emotions, or limiting beliefs that may be hindering your growth. Write them down and explore ways to release them during this phase.
- How does the Waxing Moon's energy feel in your body? Does it bring a sense of urgency, excitement, or expansion? Pay attention to how your body responds to the growing energy of this phase. Explore how you can use this physical awareness to channel your energy into productive action.

Expanding Your Waxing Moon Practice

As you work with the Waxing Moon's energy, it's essential to remember that growth is not always linear. There may be moments of great momentum and times when progress feels slower than expected. This phase encourages you to stay the course, remain adaptable, and trust that each step you take—no matter how small—is moving you toward your goals.

Here are some additional ways to expand your Waxing Moon practice:

- Movement-Based Rituals: Incorporate physical activity into your Waxing Moon rituals to embody the energy of growth and movement. Whether it's a brisk walk in nature, yoga, or dancing, engaging your body during this phase can help you feel more aligned with the lunar energy.
- Candle Magick: Light a candle to symbolize the growing light of the Waxing Moon. As the flame burns, focus on your goals and intentions, visualizing them growing brighter and stronger just like the moon.
- Crystal Work: Work with crystals that support growth and manifestation, such as citrine (for abundance and creativity), green aventurine (for opportunity and expansion), or clear quartz (for amplifying energy and intentions). Carry these crystals with you or place them on your altar during your Waxing Moon rituals.
- Herbal Baths: Take a bath infused with herbs like rosemary, peppermint, and ginger to invigorate your body and mind. As you soak in the bath, focus on how the energy of the herbs supports your personal growth and helps clear away any lingering doubts or fears.

Closing Thoughts on the Waxing Moon

The Waxing Moon is a time of action, focus, and forward momentum. It is the phase where the intentions you planted during the New Moon begin to sprout and grow. By working with the energy of the Waxing Moon, you can take deliberate, empowered steps toward manifesting your desires and bringing your goals into reality.

Remember, the journey toward manifestation requires both patience and perseverance. The energy of growth is not always immediate, but with each small action you take, you move closer to your dreams. Trust in the process, stay focused on your intentions, and allow the Waxing Moon to guide you toward your highest potential.

5

The Full Moon – Culmination, Reflection, and Release

The Full Moon is the most potent and luminous phase of the lunar cycle, representing a peak in energy, manifestation, and awareness. It is a time of culmination—when the intentions we planted during the New Moon come to fruition. The Full Moon shines its light on both our successes and challenges, allowing us to reflect on our progress, celebrate our achievements, and release what no longer serves us. In this chapter, we will explore the energy of the Full Moon, how it influences our personal growth, and how to work with herbs and rituals for reflection, healing, and release.

The Energy of the Full Moon: A Time of Completion and Illumination

The Full Moon is a powerful symbol of completion and wholeness. It represents the peak of the lunar cycle, when the moon is fully illuminated, and its energy is at its most intense. This is a time when everything is brought into the light—both the positive and the challenging aspects of our lives. The Full Moon invites us to look closely at our progress, recognize our accomplishments, and confront the things that may be holding us back.

In many spiritual traditions, the Full Moon is seen as a time of celebration, gratitude, and reflection. It is a time to acknowledge the work we have done and to express gratitude for the growth and transformation we have experienced. However, it is also a time for letting go—for releasing any limiting beliefs, patterns, or emotions that no longer align with our goals.

The energy of the Full Moon can bring heightened emotions and awareness. It illuminates the areas of our lives that need attention, making it a powerful time for healing and release. By working with the energy of the Full Moon, we can embrace the lessons we've learned, release what no longer serves us, and create space for new opportunities and growth.

How to Work with the Energy of the Full Moon

The Full Moon is an ideal time for reflection, celebration, and release. To fully harness its energy, it is important to take time to reflect on your journey, celebrate your progress, and let go of anything that is no longer aligned with your path.

Tips for Working with Full Moon Energy:

1. Reflect on Your Progress: Take time to look back on the intentions you set during the New Moon. What have you accomplished? What challenges have you faced? Reflect on your growth and acknowledge the steps you have taken toward manifesting your desires.
2. Celebrate Your Successes: The Full Moon is a time of celebration, so take a moment to honor your achievements, no matter how small. Express

gratitude for the progress you've made and the lessons you've learned along the way.

3. Release What No Longer Serves You: As the Full Moon shines its light on all aspects of your life, it may reveal areas where you are holding on to limiting beliefs, habits, or emotions. Use this time to release anything that is no longer in alignment with your goals. This could be negative thought patterns, toxic relationships, or outdated beliefs about yourself.

4. Practice Self-Care: The Full Moon can bring intense emotions to the surface, so it's important to practice self-care during this time. Take time to rest, nourish your body, and engage in activities that bring you peace and balance.

5. Express Gratitude: Gratitude is a powerful practice during the Full Moon. Take time to express thanks for the lessons, experiences, and people who have supported your growth. Gratitude opens the heart and creates space for more abundance in your life.

Herbs Associated with the Full Moon

The Full Moon is a time for reflection, healing, and release, and the herbs associated with this phase support emotional balance, purification, and spiritual clarity. These herbs can be used in teas, baths, or rituals to help you align with the energy of the Full Moon and release what no longer serves you.

• Lavender (Lavandula angustifolia): Known for its calming and soothing properties, lavender helps to ease tension and anxiety. It is an excellent herb to work with during the Full Moon, as it promotes relaxation and emotional healing. Lavender can be used in teas, essential oils, or baths to create a calming atmosphere during reflection and release.

- Sage (Salvia officinalis): Sage is a powerful cleansing herb, often used for purification and clearing negative energy. Burning sage or using it in a Full Moon bath can help cleanse your energy field and create space for new beginnings. Sage is especially useful during rituals of release, as it helps to clear away stagnant energy. If you're drawn to burning sage, remember that smudging holds sacred meaning for Indigenous cultures, and it is essential to approach this practice with respect.
- Rose (Rosa damascena): Associated with love, healing, and emotional balance, rose is a beautiful herb to work with during the Full Moon. It helps open the heart and promote self-love and compassion. Rose petals can be added to baths or teas to create a sense of peace and emotional healing.
- Chamomile (Matricaria chamomilla): Chamomile is known for its calming and soothing effects. It helps to ease stress and promote restful sleep, making it an ideal herb for the emotional intensity of the Full Moon. Drinking chamomile tea before bed can help you relax and process the emotions that arise during this phase.

Herbal Ritual for the Full Moon: Releasing and Healing Bath

This Full Moon bath ritual combines the healing and purifying properties of lavender, sage, and rose to help you release emotional blockages and create space for new growth. In addition to physical cleansing, this ritual supports emotional and energetic release, allowing you to let go of anything that may be holding you back from manifesting your intentions.

Ingredients:

- 1 tbsp dried lavender
- 1 tbsp dried rose petals
- 1 tsp dried sage

Instructions:

1. Run a warm bath and add the dried herbs to the water. As the herbs infuse the water, allow their energy to clear and cleanse your mind, body, and spirit.
2. As the herbs infuse the water, set the intention to release anything that is no longer serving you. Visualize the Full Moon's light shining down on you, illuminating any negative emotions, habits, or patterns that you are ready to let go of.
3. Soak in the bath for at least 20 minutes, allowing the herbs to cleanse and soothe your mind, body, and spirit. Let the water carry away any stagnant energy.
4. As you relax, repeat the affirmation: "I release what no longer serves me. I am open to healing and new growth."
5. When you are ready, drain the bath, imagining all of the negativity and stagnant energy being washed away with the water.

Manifestation and Reflection Prompts for the Full Moon

Use these prompts to guide your reflection and keep you focused on nurturing your intentions throughout the lunar cycle.

Manifestation Prompt:

- Take a moment to reflect on the intentions you set during the New Moon. What progress have you made? What challenges have you encountered along the way? Write down three things you are ready to release during the Full Moon—whether they are limiting beliefs, negative emotions, or old habits. Reflect on how letting go of these things will create space for new opportunities and growth.

Reflection Prompts:

- What has come to fruition in my life since the New Moon? How can I celebrate my achievements, no matter how big or small?
- What am I ready to release—emotionally, mentally, or physically—so that I can create space for new energy and experiences?
- How have I grown or evolved since setting my intentions, and what lessons have I learned during this cycle?

Journaling Prompts:

- Reflect on your journey from the New Moon to the Full Moon. Write down three things you are proud of accomplishing and any unexpected results that arose.
- What are you holding onto that no longer serves you? Write down the emotions, habits, or limiting beliefs that you're ready to let go of.
- How does the Full Moon's energy feel in your body? Does it bring a sense of completion, tension, or relief? Explore how your body responds to this energetic peak.

Expanding Your Full Moon Practice

While the Full Moon is often associated with reflection and release, there are various ways to deepen your connection with this phase to fully harness its power. This is a time of intense energy, emotional clarity, and heightened awareness, making it a rich period for both celebration and letting go. By working with the moon's energy consciously, you can engage in a variety of practices that help release what no longer serves you and embrace your full potential.

Here are some additional ways to expand your Full Moon practice:

- Moonlight Meditation: If possible, find a quiet outdoor space where you can sit under the Full Moon's light. As you meditate, allow the moon's energy to illuminate your thoughts and emotions. Focus on your breath, and imagine the moonlight filling your body with healing energy. Let it cleanse and clear away any tension or emotional blocks.

- Fire Ritual for Release: Fire is a powerful element for transformation, and performing a burning ritual during the Full Moon is a potent way to release negative energy or limiting beliefs. Write down on a piece of paper the things you wish to let go of—fears, doubts, bad habits, or emotional baggage. Safely burn the paper in a fireproof dish or outside, visualizing those things being transmuted into positive energy and leaving your life for good.

- Candle Magick for Gratitude: Choose a white or silver candle to represent the illumination and completion of the Full Moon. As you light the candle, focus on all the things you are grateful for in your life. Reflect on the progress you've made, and express gratitude for the lessons, growth, and support you've experienced. Allow the candle to burn as a symbol of your gratitude and acceptance of your journey.

- Crystal Work: Work with crystals that resonate with the energy of release, reflection, and balance. Clear quartz (for amplification), selenite (for cleansing), and amethyst (for emotional balance) are excellent companions during the Full Moon. Place these crystals on your altar or carry them with you as you release and reflect.

- Full Moon Water: Similar to the New Moon, the Full Moon is a perfect time to charge water with lunar energy. Place a jar of water outside or by a window under the Full Moon's light, letting it absorb the moon's energy. Use this water in future rituals, baths, or even as a cleansing mist to refresh your space or energy field.

Closing Thoughts on the Full Moon

The Full Moon is a sacred time for reflection, celebration, and release. It is a time when the moon's light illuminates everything—both the achievements and the areas where we still have work to do. This illumination allows us to see clearly and make empowered choices about what to keep and what to release as we move forward.

By consciously working with the Full Moon, you can create a powerful practice of personal growth and transformation. The energy of this phase encourages us to celebrate the progress we've made, acknowledge the challenges we've faced, and let go of anything that no longer aligns with our highest good. The Full Moon invites us to take a deep breath, honor our journey, and trust in the ongoing cycles of growth and renewal.

As you embrace the energy of the Full Moon, remember that release is an essential part of the process of manifestation. By letting go of what no longer serves you, you create space for new opportunities, insights, and growth. Trust in the wisdom of the moon's cycles, and know that with each phase, you are continuously evolving, healing, and moving toward your fullest potential.

6

The Waning Moon – Reflection, Release, and Renewal

As the Full Moon begins to wane, the energy of the lunar cycle shifts from growth and action to reflection, release, and renewal. The Waning Moon, which includes the Waning Gibbous, Last Quarter, and Waning Crescent phases, is a time of slowing down, turning inward, and letting go. This is when we are invited to assess what has served us well during the cycle and what we need to release in order to create space for new opportunities in the future. In this chapter, we will explore how to work with the energy of the Waning Moon, the herbs that support this phase, and how to embrace the natural process of release and renewal.

The Energy of the Waning Moon: A Time of Surrender and Reflection

The Waning Moon represents the process of decline and release. As the moon's light diminishes, we are called to reflect on the experiences, lessons, and emotions that have surfaced during the lunar cycle. This is a time for letting go of anything that no longer serves our highest good—whether that's emotional baggage, limiting beliefs, unhealthy habits, or even relationships that are out of alignment.

Just as the moon transitions from its peak of illumination during the Full Moon to the darkness of the New Moon, we too are invited to move through a process of release and surrender. This phase is often associated with rest, recovery, and renewal, as we shed what no longer serves us and prepare for a fresh start with the next New Moon.

In many spiritual traditions, the Waning Moon is seen as a time for introspection, healing, and closure. It's a time to release the burdens we've been carrying and create space for new beginnings. Whether it's letting go of a project, a relationship, or a mindset, the energy of the Waning Moon supports us in this process of release and transformation.

How to Work with the Energy of the Waning Moon

The Waning Moon invites us to slow down, reflect on our journey, and release what is no longer in alignment with our intentions. By consciously working with this energy, we can experience deep emotional and spiritual renewal, clearing the path for new growth in the next lunar cycle.

Tips for Working with Waning Moon Energy:

1. Reflect on the Cycle: Take time to reflect on the journey of the current lunar cycle. What have you accomplished? What challenges have you faced? What lessons have you learned? Use this phase to gain insight into your personal growth.
2. Release What No Longer Serves You: The Waning Moon is a time for release. Whether it's a limiting belief, a habit, or an emotion that's been weighing you down, this phase offers the perfect opportunity to let go of what's holding you back. You might find it helpful to write down what you wish to release and then perform a symbolic act of letting go, such as burning the paper or burying it in the earth.
3. Practice Self-Care and Rest: The Waning Moon is a time for rest and recovery. Allow yourself to slow down, recharge, and reflect. Engage in practices that nurture your mind, body, and spirit, such as journaling, meditation, or gentle movement.
4. Prepare for Renewal: As you release what no longer serves you, you are creating space for new possibilities. Use this time to prepare for the fresh start that the New Moon will bring. Visualize the new energy, opportunities, and experiences you want to invite into your life.

Herbs Associated with the Waning Moon

The herbs associated with the Waning Moon are those that support emotional release, purification, and deep reflection. These herbs help to cleanse the mind and spirit, facilitate emotional healing, and promote rest and renewal. They can be used in teas, baths, or rituals to support the process of letting go.

- Mugwort (Artemisia vulgaris): Known for its ability to enhance intuition and promote deep reflection, mugwort is a powerful herb for the Waning Moon. It helps to bring subconscious emotions to the surface and supports the process of release and healing. Mugwort can be used in teas or burned as incense during rituals of release.
- Juniper (Juniperus communis): Juniper is often associated with purification and protection. It helps to clear negative energy and supports emotional release. Burning juniper or using it in a cleansing bath can help you let go of stagnant energy and create space for new beginnings.
- Mint (Mentha spp.): Mint is a refreshing and uplifting herb that helps to clear mental fog and promote emotional clarity. It can be used in teas or baths to help release emotional blockages and refresh the mind and spirit.
- Skullcap (Scutellaria lateriflora): Skullcap is a calming herb that supports relaxation and emotional balance. It is often used to ease anxiety, promote restful sleep, and soothe the nervous system. Skullcap tea is a wonderful way to unwind and reflect during the Waning Moon.

Herbal Ritual for the Waning Moon: Releasing and Renewing Tea

This herbal tea blend combines the reflective and purifying properties of mugwort, juniper, and skullcap to support the process of release and renewal during the Waning Moon. This tea can be enjoyed during a quiet moment of reflection as you let go of what no longer serves you.

Ingredients:

- 1 tsp dried mugwort
- 1 tsp dried skullcap

- ½ tsp dried mint
- ½ tsp dried juniper berries

Instructions:

1. Boil a cup of water and add the herbs.
2. Let steep for 10 minutes.
3. Strain and drink while reflecting on what you are ready to release.
4. As you sip your tea, repeat the affirmation: "I release all that no longer serves me. I create space for healing and renewal."

This simple ritual will help you align with the Waning Moon's energy, making space for emotional release and personal growth.

Manifestation and Reflection Prompts for the Waning Moon

Use these prompts to guide your reflection and keep you focused on nurturing your intentions throughout the lunar cycle.

Manifestation Prompt:

- Take a moment to reflect on the lessons and experiences of this lunar cycle. What are you ready to release? Write down three things you wish to let go of during this Waning Moon phase—whether they are limiting beliefs, emotions, or habits. Reflect on how letting go of these things will create space for new growth and opportunities in the next cycle.

Reflection Prompts:

- What patterns or habits have surfaced that I am ready to shed as I enter this phase of release and renewal?
- How can I use this time to reflect on my personal growth, and what do I need to let go of to continue evolving?
- What am I doing to nourish my mind, body, and spirit during this quieter, introspective phase of the lunar cycle?

Expanded Journaling Prompts:

- Write about one area of your life where you feel resistance to change. How can you gently release that resistance and invite healing?
- What has come up during this lunar cycle that needs further reflection? Write about any emotions or insights that have surfaced.
- Imagine yourself one month from now—what do you hope to have released and healed by then? Write down what your future self looks like after embracing renewal.

Expanding Your Waning Moon Practices

The Waning Moon offers a unique opportunity to deepen your spiritual and emotional practices by focusing on release, reflection, and renewal. While many people think of release as simply letting go, the Waning Moon encourages us to dig deeper into what it means to consciously surrender and clear the path for new growth. Below are suggestions for expanding your practice during this phase.

1. Journaling: For Deep Emotional Release During the Waning Moon, make journaling a daily practice of introspection and emotional release. Rather than just writing about your surface-level feelings, ask yourself deeper questions about what you are ready to let go of emotionally. Use prompts such as "What fears am I holding onto that no longer serve my growth?" "What relationships or situations bring me stress, and why do I continue to engage with them?" "How can I lovingly release past versions of myself that are no longer aligned with my current path?" This deeper level of self-inquiry can reveal limiting beliefs and patterns that have been operating under the surface and will help you consciously choose what to release.

2. Physical Decluttering As a Reflection of Internal Release: Incorporate the concept of physical decluttering into your Waning Moon practice. As you release emotional and mental baggage, you can mirror this by decluttering your physical space. Begin with areas that feel heavy, chaotic, or overwhelming, such as closets, drawers, or your workspace. As you clear physical items, visualize yourself releasing stagnant energy from your life. You might ask yourself: "What do I hold onto physically that no longer brings me joy or serves a purpose?" "How does my external environment reflect my internal state, and how can I clear both?" This act of cleansing your surroundings can offer a tangible way to embrace release and welcome clarity.

3. Daily Meditation For Release and Surrender: Meditation is an essential practice during the Waning Moon. Incorporating guided meditations or silent reflection focusing on release and surrender can help anchor your energy. Create a daily habit of spending a few minutes in meditation, visualizing any tension, worries, or stagnant emotions leaving your body with each exhale. You may want to use a mantra such as, "I surrender to the flow of life," or "I release all that no longer serves me." To deepen your practice, consider focusing on a specific chakra (energy center) during your meditation. The Root Chakra (Muladhara) or the Heart Chakra (Anahata) are ideal focal points for grounding and emotional release during this phase.

4. Herbal Baths and Rituals for Release: To complement the bath ritual outlined earlier, consider incorporating a weekly or bi-weekly bath during the Waning Moon that focuses specifically on emotional release and energetic cleansing. Enhance the experience with a salt scrub made from Epsom salt, lavender oil, and peppermint for renewal and clarity. Additionally, consider conducting a Waning Moon Candle Ritual: Candle Ritual: Take a black candle (symbolizing release) and inscribe it with words or symbols representing what you wish to let go of. As the candle burns, sit in silence and meditate on the areas of your life that require release. Visualize those energies dissolving with the flame, making space for new energy in the next lunar cycle.

5. Nature Walks for Reflective Clarity: Spending time in nature is especially powerful during the Waning Moon. Engage in mindful walking, tuning into the natural cycles of decay, rest, and renewal around you. Observe the changing seasons, leaves falling, or the stillness of a forest. This can be a symbolic reminder of the beauty and necessity of release. As you walk, reflect on:*"What lessons can I learn from nature's cycles of release?" "How can I mimic nature's ability to let go without resistance?"* Use these walks to deepen your connection to the natural world while honoring your own process of reflection.

6. Moon Phase Affirmations for Surrender: Incorporating affirmations is a powerful way to align with the energies of the Waning Moon. Begin your mornings or close your evenings with affirmations such as: *"I honor the wisdom of release." "I trust the process of letting go to create space for renewal." "I welcome the calm and clarity that follows surrender."* These affirmations help reinforce the mindset of releasing with grace, empowering you to embrace the flow of the lunar cycles and your own internal rhythm of growth and reflection.

Closing Thoughts on Expanding Your Waning Moon Practice

The Waning Moon is a sacred time for deep personal reflection, emotional surrender, and the mindful release of everything that no longer serves your higher purpose. By expanding your practices during this phase, you allow yourself the space to evolve without holding onto the baggage that has weighed you down.

The moon's quiet retreat into darkness reminds us that release is not an ending but rather a necessary part of the cycle that makes way for new beginnings. Through these rituals, reflections, and affirmations, you can create a deeper, more intentional relationship with your own process of letting go, ensuring that each new cycle of the moon brings you closer to the growth and fulfillment you seek.

7

Lunar Eclipses and Blue Moons - Harnessing Rare Energies

Lunar eclipses and blue moons are rare and powerful celestial events that heighten the moon's energy, offering unique opportunities for transformation, revelation, and manifestation. These phenomena stand apart from the regular lunar phases, presenting potent moments for personal and spiritual growth. Their energy can feel intense, but it's exactly this intensity that makes them prime opportunities for deep reflection, release, and rapid shifts in our lives. In this chapter, we will delve into the magick of lunar eclipses and blue moons, explore the herbs and rituals that align with these transformative energies, and discover how to work with them for profound healing and growth.

The Energy of Lunar Eclipses: Sudden Shifts and Revelations

A lunar eclipse occurs when the Earth passes between the sun and the moon, casting a shadow over the moon's surface. This cosmic alignment symbolizes a moment of interruption—a pause in the usual flow of light and energy. Eclipses are moments of intensified energy and sudden shifts, revealing deep truths and stirring emotions that may have been hidden from conscious awareness. Unlike the steady progression of the moon's phases, eclipses bring abrupt changes, and with them, powerful opportunities for transformation.

Lunar eclipses are often seen as cosmic resets, bringing to the surface patterns, emotions, or situations that need attention. These revelations can be uncomfortable but are necessary for our growth and healing. During a lunar eclipse, we are asked to look deeply within ourselves and address the shadow aspects of our being—the fears, doubts, or unresolved issues that keep us stuck in old patterns.

While lunar eclipses may feel overwhelming, they are not to be feared. They are moments of accelerated change, clearing the way for breakthroughs and new beginnings. Eclipses bring about rapid endings and beginnings, often speeding up the natural progression of our lives in ways we may not have anticipated. This energy can feel intense, but it ultimately serves our highest good by pushing us toward greater alignment and truth.

How to Harness the Energy of a Lunar Eclipse

Lunar eclipses are prime times for shadow work—diving into the hidden, darker aspects of the self. They provide an opportunity to confront those parts of our psyche that we typically avoid. Working with the energy of a lunar eclipse requires courage, openness, and a willingness to embrace change.

Tips for Harnessing Lunar Eclipse Energy:

1. Shadow Work: Use this time to explore the shadow aspects of yourself. Journaling, deep meditation, or seeking guidance from a therapist or

healer can be powerful ways to engage with this practice. Ask yourself: "What fears, wounds, or limiting beliefs have been operating in the background of my life?"

2. Release Rituals: Eclipses are ideal for performing rituals focused on release. Write down what you are ready to let go of—whether it's a toxic relationship, a self-limiting belief, or an emotional pattern. Burn the paper or bury it in the earth as a symbolic act of release.

3. Embrace Change: Eclipses often bring swift changes, some of which may be unexpected. Practice surrender by accepting the shifts that occur during this time. Trust that the universe is clearing out what no longer serves you, making room for growth and renewal.

4. Grounding Practices: The energy of a lunar eclipse can feel chaotic and intense, making grounding essential. Spend time in nature, walk barefoot on the earth, or practice grounding visualizations to stay centered during this powerful time.

Herbs Associated with Lunar Eclipses

The herbs associated with lunar eclipses facilitate emotional release, grounding, and shadow work. These herbs help us process the intensity of eclipse energy and support our emotional and spiritual well-being.

- Valerian (Valeriana officinalis): A deeply calming herb, valerian is used to ease anxiety and promote relaxation. During a lunar eclipse, valerian helps to soothe the nervous system, making it easier to navigate heightened emotions and revelations.
- Mugwort (Artemisia vulgaris): Mugwort is a powerful herb for intuition, dream work, and shadow exploration. It helps bring hidden emotions and subconscious patterns to the surface, making it a valuable ally during

lunar eclipses.

- Ashwagandha (Withania somnifera): An adaptogen that supports stress management and emotional resilience, ashwagandha helps us stay grounded during intense shifts. It stabilizes the mind and body during transformative times.

Herbal Ritual for a Lunar Eclipse: Shadow Work Tea

This tea blend supports the process of shadow work, helping you explore and release hidden aspects of yourself during a lunar eclipse.

Ingredients:

- 1 tsp dried valerian root
- 1 tsp dried mugwort
- ½ tsp dried ashwagandha

Instructions:

1. Boil a cup of water and add the herbs.
2. Let steep for 10 minutes.
3. Strain and drink while reflecting on any emotions or patterns that have surfaced during the eclipse.
4. As you sip your tea, repeat the affirmation:

"I release what no longer serves me. I trust the process of transformation."

The Energy of Blue Moons: Rare Opportunities and Manifestation

A blue moon occurs when there are two full moons within a single calendar month or four full moons in a single season, making it a rare celestial event. The phrase "once in a blue moon" reflects this rarity and the unique power these moons hold. The energy of a blue moon is associated with abundance, manifestation, and amplified potential, making it a time for bold action and confident pursuit of long-term goals.

Blue moons are considered windows of opportunity, offering a chance to align with the energies of expansion, abundance, and achievement. These are the moments when the universe is especially responsive to our desires, and the veil between the spiritual and material worlds is thin. The energy of a blue moon magnifies our intentions, making it an ideal time to focus on large-scale projects, life changes, or any dream that requires a leap of faith.

How to Harness the Energy of a Blue Moon

The energy of a blue moon is expansive and filled with possibility. It's a time to dream big, take risks, and step fully into your power. Blue moons are moments of heightened manifestation potential, and they offer a unique opportunity to pursue long-held dreams with confidence and clarity.

Tips for Harnessing Blue Moon Energy:

1. Set Bold Intentions: Use the energy of a blue moon to set intentions for long-term goals. Be specific, clear, and ambitious. This is a time to think big—write down what you want to manifest over the coming months or years.
2. Take Action: A blue moon is a time for bold moves. Whether it's launching a new project, taking a risk, or stepping out of your comfort zone, the energy of a blue moon supports taking confident action toward your dreams.
3. Trust in Abundance: The energy of a blue moon is abundant and expansive. Trust that the universe is supporting you and that your desires are within reach. Visualize yourself receiving the abundance you seek and practice gratitude for the blessings you are manifesting.
4. Work with Amplifying Herbs: Herbs such as basil and cinnamon are ideal for amplifying manifestation energy. Use them in teas, baths, or rituals to enhance your intentions and align with the abundant energy of the blue moon.

Herbs Associated with Blue Moons

The herbs associated with blue moons amplify energy, abundance, and manifestation. These herbs help to magnify your intentions and align your energy with the expansive potential of the blue moon.

- Basil (Ocimum basilicum): A symbol of abundance and prosperity, basil amplifies positive energy and enhances manifestation. It can be used in teas, baths, or as an offering during rituals to attract prosperity.

- Cinnamon (Cinnamomum verum): A warming and energizing herb, cinnamon boosts motivation and manifestation. It is often used in spells for abundance and success.
- Dandelion (Taraxacum officinale): Associated with wishes and resilience, dandelion helps strengthen your intentions and align your energy with the universe's abundance.

Herbal Ritual for a Blue Moon: Abundance and Manifestation Bath

This ritual bath combines the amplifying energies of basil, cinnamon, and dandelion to support manifestation during a blue moon. Use this bath to set bold intentions and align with the energy of abundance.

Ingredients:

- 1 tbsp dried basil
- 1 tsp ground cinnamon
- 1 tbsp dried dandelion leaves

Instructions:

1. Run a warm bath and add the herbs to the water.
2. As you soak, visualize your intentions coming to fruition. Focus on the areas in your life where you seek abundance and growth.

3. See yourself surrounded by golden light, symbolizing the abundant energy of the blue moon.
4. As you soak, repeat the affirmation:

"I am open to abundance. I manifest my desires with confidence and trust."

5.Stay in the bath for at least 20 minutes, allowing the herbs and the energy of the blue moon to infuse your body and spirit with their magnifying power.

Expanding Your Lunar Eclipse and Blue Moon Practices

To truly harness the rare energies of lunar eclipses and blue moons, it's important to explore a variety of rituals, meditations, and practices that can deepen your connection to these powerful moments. These events offer potent energies that can accelerate transformation and magnify manifestations, making them ideal times for engaging in more profound spiritual work.

Expanded Practices for Lunar Eclipses

1. Lunar Eclipse Meditation for Release and Transformation: Eclipses often bring hidden truths to the surface, and meditating during a lunar eclipse can help you uncover and release deep-seated emotional blockages. Set aside 15-30 minutes for this practice:Find a quiet, comfortable space. Light a candle or burn mugwort or sage to purify the space. Close your eyes, take several deep breaths, and visualize the shadow of the Earth moving across the moon. As the shadow passes, imagine your own hidden fears, limiting beliefs, or unresolved emotions surfacing. Allow them to come to the forefront of your mind. With each exhale, visualize releasing these blockages, allowing the moon's transformative energy to clear them away. Close the meditation by expressing gratitude for the

lessons revealed by the eclipse, knowing that this release is preparing you for new growth.

2. Eclipse Shadow Work Ritual: Since lunar eclipses are perfect for shadow work, you can use this practice to explore the hidden or neglected parts of your psyche: Set up your sacred space with a black or dark blue candle to represent the shadow aspect. Write down any recurring patterns, fears, or emotional blocks that have been revealed to you recently. In a journal, explore these areas more deeply, asking yourself how these patterns affect your life, and what lessons they might be teaching you. Once you've processed your reflections, consider burning the paper to symbolically release these shadows into the universe, allowing for transformation.

3. Journaling for Eclipse Revelations: Lunar eclipses often bring revelations or epiphanies. Use this time to journal deeply about what is being illuminated in your life: What has come to the surface during this eclipse that you haven't been willing to face before? What patterns or behaviors are you ready to release? How can you step into a more aligned version of yourself after this eclipse? This practice allows you to fully embrace the lessons of the eclipse and consciously integrate them into your life.

Expanded Practices for Blue Moons

1. Manifestation Candle Ritual: Blue moons are a time for amplifying your manifestations and setting bold intentions. This ritual uses the power of a blue moon to magnify your desires: Choose a candle that represents your goal (gold or green for abundance, pink for love, blue for healing, etc.). Write your intentions clearly on a piece of paper. Be as specific as possible, focusing on what you wish to manifest over the coming months. Anoint the candle with basil or cinnamon oil, and light it with the intention of amplifying your desire. As the candle burns, visualize your goals coming to fruition. See yourself living your dream and feel

the emotions of having already achieved it. Once the candle has burned down, keep the intention paper in a safe place until the next blue moon, when you can revisit your progress.

2. Vision Boarding for Blue Moon Manifestation: A blue moon's rare energy offers the perfect opportunity to create or update a vision board. This visual representation of your goals and desires allows you to harness the amplified potential of the blue moon. Gather magazines, images, words, or other materials that resonate with your long-term goals. Create a board that visually represents your dreams and desires, focusing on areas such as career, relationships, health, personal growth, and travel. As you place each image or word on the board, state aloud what it represents and how you intend to manifest it. Hang the board somewhere you can see it daily, allowing it to serve as a reminder of the blue moon's energy supporting your manifestation journey.

3. Prosperity Bath Ritual: Amplify your abundance using the potent energies of a blue moon with this prosperity bath: Prepare a bath infused with basil, cinnamon, and dandelion, and a few drops of prosperity oil if available. As you soak in the bath, visualize yourself surrounded by golden light, representing wealth, success, and abundance in all areas of your life. Focus on the specific ways you want abundance to manifest, whether in your career, relationships, or personal growth. Affirm to yourself: "I am open to abundance. I welcome prosperity in all its forms." After your bath, write down any insights or inspirations that came up during the ritual, reinforcing your intentions.

Moonstone and Crystals in Eclipse and Blue Moon Rituals

Working with moonstone or other crystals can enhance the impact of lunar eclipse and blue moon rituals. Moonstone, in particular, is aligned with lunar energies and can help amplify your intuitive abilities and connection to the moon. Other crystals, such as clear quartz for amplification or black tourmaline for grounding, can be placed on your altar or held during rituals to enhance your practice.

Closing Thoughts on Lunar Eclipses and Blue Moons

Lunar eclipses and blue moons offer some of the most powerful opportunities for transformation, healing, and manifestation. By working with the energy of these rare celestial events, you can experience profound shifts in your personal growth and spiritual journey. Whether you are releasing old patterns during a lunar eclipse or amplifying your intentions during a blue moon, these moments provide an opening for deep healing and expansion.

As you continue to engage with the moon's cycles, remember to approach each phase with openness, intention, and trust in the process. These rare events can bring unexpected revelations, but they always guide you toward a deeper alignment with your highest self. Embrace the opportunities they offer, and let the energies of the moon support you in your ongoing evolution.

8

Lunar Alignment: Harmonizing Mind and Body with the Moon

The connection between the moon's cycles and our mental and emotional well-being is a relationship that stretches back to ancient times. Across cultures, the moon has been a symbol of reflection, transformation, and healing. Today, science and holistic practices continue to affirm the moon's profound influence on our physical and mental health. By aligning our personal rhythms with the moon's phases and incorporating herbs into our daily practices, we can cultivate a deeper sense of harmony, balance, and well-being.

In this chapter, we will explore how to work with the moon's cycles to support mental health, how specific herbs can enhance emotional and mental clarity, and how to integrate rituals that harmonize mind and body with lunar energy.

The Power of Living in Sync with Nature's Cycles

Humans have long recognized that their bodies and minds are influenced by the natural world. From circadian rhythms tied to the sun to hormonal cycles connected to the moon, our bodies are attuned to the Earth's natural movements. Living in sync with these cycles allows us to move through life with greater flow, avoiding the stress and burnout that comes from pushing against the natural ebb and flow of energy.

For mental health, aligning with the moon is particularly beneficial because it provides a structured way to manage our emotional highs and lows. Just as the moon moves from dark to light and back again, we too experience times of growth, intensity, release, and renewal. Recognizing these internal cycles allows us to address mental and emotional challenges at the appropriate times and with the proper support.

How the Moon Affects Mental Health

The relationship between lunar cycles and mental health has been acknowl-edged for centuries. Some studies even suggest that the moon's gravitational pull and its influence on water can affect human emotions and behaviors. Ancient civilizations believed that mental health, especially conditions like anxiety or depression, could be influenced by the moon, a belief echoed by the term "lunacy," which originates from the Latin word luna, meaning moon.

From a modern perspective, the moon's phases can serve as a guide for when to engage in certain types of mental and emotional self-care. During the New Moon, we can set intentions for emotional growth. As the moon waxes, we can focus on building new habits or pursuing therapy. The Full Moon, with its heightened energy, can be a time for emotional release, and the Waning Moon allows for reflection and rest.

By being mindful of the moon's phases, we can proactively manage our mental health, allowing time for recovery, renewal, and self-discovery.

How to Incorporate Lunar Cycles into Mental Health Practices

Each lunar phase offers unique opportunities to support mental health. By understanding the emotional energy of each phase, we can tailor our mental health practices accordingly. Below is a breakdown of how each moon phase impacts mental well-being, along with recommended herbal rituals to enhance the process.

New Moon: Beginnings and Intention-Setting

The New Moon marks the beginning of the lunar cycle, offering a time for setting intentions and creating a foundation for emotional and mental well-being. During this time, we feel a sense of quiet and stillness, making it ideal for introspection, self-reflection, and goal-setting.

Mental Health Focus:

During the New Moon, focus on creating clarity and setting achievable mental health goals. Whether you're starting a new practice like mindfulness medi tation, developing a self-care routine, or addressing emotional challenges, this phase supports fresh beginnings.

Herbal Ritual for the New Moon:

Create a tea blend that encourages mental clarity and emotional balance. Use calming herbs like chamomile and skullcap, which promote relaxation and help alleviate anxiety.

- Ingredients: 1 tsp dried chamomile, 1 tsp dried skullcap

- Instructions: Boil a cup of water and steep the herbs for 10 minutes. As you sip, reflect on your mental health goals for the coming cycle. Repeat the affirmation: "I open myself to new beginnings and mental clarity."

Waxing Moon: Growth and Action

As the moon grows in light during the Waxing phase, it symbolizes a time of action, momentum, and growth. This is when we take the steps needed to bring our intentions into reality.

Mental Health Focus:

During the Waxing Moon, focus on building mental resilience and taking active steps toward emotional healing. This is the phase for practicing mindfulness, setting boundaries, or engaging in new therapeutic techniques. It's a time to build confidence and work on mental fortitude.

Herbal Ritual for the Waxing Moon:

Create an energizing herbal tonic to support focus and mental strength. Adaptogenic herbs like gotu kola and ginseng help promote sustained energy, mental clarity, and focus.

- Ingredients: 1 tsp dried gotu kola, 1 tsp ginseng root
- Instructions: Boil a cup of water and steep the herbs for 10 minutes. As you drink, visualize yourself taking steady steps toward your goals. Affirm: "I am focused, energized, and moving forward with confidence."

Full Moon: Reflection and Release

The Full Moon represents the peak of emotional energy. It is a time of illumination, reflection, and culmination. During this phase, emotions are heightened, making it an ideal time to release stress, anxiety, or lingering emotional blockages.

Mental Health Focus:

The Full Moon can be a time of emotional overwhelm for some, but it also offers an opportunity for deep reflection and healing. This phase encourages us to confront unresolved emotions, reflect on our progress, and let go of anything that is no longer serving our mental health.

Herbal Ritual for the Full Moon:

Create a calming bath using lavender and rose petals, herbs known for their emotional soothing properties. This bath ritual will help calm heightened emotions and support emotional release.

- Ingredients: 1 tbsp dried lavender, 1 tbsp dried rose petals
- Instructions: Add the herbs to a warm bath and soak for at least 20 minutes. As you relax, imagine the Full Moon illuminating your emotional landscape, allowing you to release stress and embrace emotional healing. Affirm: "I release what no longer serves me and embrace emotional healing."

Waning Moon: Reflection, Release, and Renewal

As the moon's light begins to fade, the Waning Moon represents a time for slowing down, introspection, and release. It encourages us to let go of emotional baggage and make room for new possibilities in the next cycle.

Mental Health Focus:

Use the Waning Moon to focus on mental and emotional release. This is a time to reflect on your progress and identify patterns or thoughts that may be holding you back. Release old habits, negative self-talk, or stress that no longer serves you, and allow space for renewal and rest.

Herbal Ritual for the Waning Moon:

Create a tea with mugwort and lemon balm to aid in emotional release and renewal. Mugwort helps with reflection, while lemon balm supports calm and emotional recovery.

- Ingredients: 1 tsp dried mugwort, 1 tsp dried lemon balm
- Instructions: Boil a cup of water and steep the herbs for 10 minutes. As you sip the tea, reflect on what you are ready to release and let go of emotionally. Affirm: "I release old patterns and embrace emotional renewal."

Incorporating Herbs and Mental Health Practices

In addition to lunar alignment, herbs play a key role in supporting mental health. Herbs can be used to soothe stress, promote emotional balance, and facilitate mental clarity. Regularly incorporating herbal teas, baths, and tinctures into your daily routine helps build a stronger foundation for emotional resilience and mental clarity.

1. Herbal Teas:

Drink herbal teas that support your mental health goals in alignment with the lunar phases. Use calming herbs like chamomile during the New Moon, energizing herbs like ginseng during the Waxing phase, and cleansing herbs like sage or mugwort during the Waning phase.

2. Herbal Baths:

Add calming herbs like lavender or rose to your bath during the Full Moon to release tension and stress. The warmth of the water combined with the soothing properties of the herbs creates a powerful ritual for emotional healing.

3. Herbal Smudging:

Burn sage, rosemary, or mugwort during meditation or rituals. These herbs help cleanse your mental space, inviting a sense of clarity and peace.

4. Essential Oils and Tinctures:

Use lavender oil for stress relief, or take valerian or lemon balm tinctures to calm the nervous system during moments of mental or emotional overwhelm.

Recap of Lunar Phases and Herbs for Mental Health

In this chapter, we have explored how the moon's phases influence mental and emotional well-being, and how you can align your mental health practices with each phase. By working with herbs that correspond to each lunar phase, you can enhance your ability to manage stress, gain clarity, and heal emotionally.

- New Moon: Chamomile and skullcap for clarity and intention-setting.
- Waxing Moon: Gotu kola and ginseng for focus and action.
- Full Moon: Lavender and rose petals for reflection and emotional release.
- Waning Moon: Mugwort and lemon balm for emotional healing and renewal.

By aligning with the moon's phases and using the natural healing power of herbs, you can create a balanced and holistic approach to mental health that supports emotional growth, healing, and resilience.

9

The Intersection of Science, Spirit, and Holistic Healing with the Moon

For centuries, humanity has turned to the moon as a guide for emotional balance, spiritual growth, and physical well-being. The moon's rhythmic dance has been a source of inspiration in rituals, healing practices, and agricultural cycles. But beyond ancient traditions, modern science supports the idea that the moon's influence extends to our biology and mental health, adding a layer of credibility and depth to our spiritual practices.

In this chapter, we bridge ancient wisdom from systems like Ayurveda, Traditional Chinese Medicine (TCM), and Western holistic medicine with modern science to explore how lunar phases affect human biology and mental health. Through credible case studies and personal experiences, we demonstrate how aligning with the moon's cycles can lead to lasting and tangible healing in our lives.

The Moon's Influence on Human Biology: An Ancient and Modern Perspective

The connection between the moon and human biology has been observed and studied across different cultures for thousands of years. From ancient Vedic scholars in India to Chinese Taoists, the moon's energy was seen as a force that influenced everything from human fertility to the growth of plants and the flow of energy within the body.

Lunar Rhythms in Ayurveda:

In Ayurvedic traditions, the moon is linked to the principle of Kapha—one of the three doshas that represent bodily humors. Kapha energy is cooling, nurturing, and reflective, qualities deeply connected to the moon. In Ayurveda, the lunar cycles are believed to influence emotional well-being, fertility, and mental clarity. Practices like Chandra Namaskar (moon salutation) are designed to align the body's energy with the moon's gentle and cooling influence. Ayurvedic physicians often recommend aligning herbal treatments and detoxification practices with the waning moon to support the natural process of release.

Traditional Chinese Medicine (TCM):

In TCM, the moon is associated with the yin energy—representing the passive, receptive, and nourishing forces in the body. The waxing moon is viewed as a time when yang (active energy) builds, while the waning moon promotes yin nourishment and reflection. Acupuncturists align certain treatments with the moon's phases, especially focusing on harmonizing yin and yang energy during full or new moons. Herbs like schisandra and dong quai are used in TCM to balance reproductive and emotional health in sync with lunar cycles.

Western Science and Circadian Biology:

In recent decades, Western science has explored how the moon's cycles impact circadian rhythms—the body's internal clock. Studies show that the moon's gravitational pull can influence human sleep patterns, hormone regulation, and even mood shifts. These natural cycles are vital to mental health and are increasingly recognized in holistic medicine.

A 2013 study published in Current Biology found that during the Full Moon, participants took longer to fall asleep and experienced less deep sleep. This disruption, linked to changes in melatonin production, highlights how lunar rhythms subtly impact our biological processes, affecting both our mental and physical health.

Case Study: The Full Moon and Sleep Quality

A 2014 study published in Sleep Medicine analyzed the impact of lunar cycles on sleep patterns over a three-month period. Participants who were monitored using polysomnography reported that during the Full Moon, sleep disturbances were common, with reduced deep sleep and overall poorer sleep quality. Many participants also noted increased emotional sensitivity and a heightened awareness of unresolved stressors during the Full Moon, illustrating the moon's potential to influence not only physical rest but also emotional health.

Hormonal Cycles and the Moon

The connection between the moon and human reproductive health has been noted across various cultures, especially regarding menstrual cycles. In ancient times, women's menstrual cycles were thought to synchronize with the lunar phases. Today, while direct scientific evidence on this link is inconclusive, many holistic practices acknowledge that the moon's energy plays a role in regulating emotional and hormonal health.

Ayurveda's View on Women's Cycles:

In Ayurveda, the moon's cooling and reflective energy is considered essential for women's reproductive health. Herbal treatments for hormonal balance, such as those using shatavari or ashoka, are often aligned with the moon's phases, particularly during the New Moon and Full Moon. These herbs are believed to restore hormonal equilibrium and support emotional well-being.

Traditional Chinese Medicine and Reproductive Health:

TCM practitioners observe that the body's energetic balance—between yin and yang—influences fertility and reproductive health. The Full Moon, representing the peak of yin, is believed to be a powerful time for conception. TCM herbs like angelica (known as dong quai) and white peony are used during this time to nourish blood and support the liver's role in hormone regulation.

Case Study: Hormone Synchronization and the Moon

Dr. Charlotte Helfrich-Förster conducted a study in 2021 examining the connection between lunar cycles and menstrual synchronization. Her research revealed that women's menstrual cycles sometimes aligned with the moon's phases, especially when exposed to natural light. This synchronization, most common in women with minimal exposure to artificial light, suggests that the moon's gravitational pull might influence hormonal fluctuations, particularly those regulated by melatonin and serotonin.

The Moon and Mental Health

Emotional and mental health have long been linked to the lunar phases. Ancient cultures believed that mental states fluctuated with the waxing and waning of the moon. Today, science recognizes that our emotions, stress levels, and even psychiatric disorders can be affected by these natural rhythms.

Ancient Views on Lunar Influence:

In both Ayurvedic and Chinese medicine, emotional health is seen as deeply connected to the lunar cycle. The waxing moon builds energy, increasing stress or anxiety in some individuals, while the waning moon allows for emotional release and introspection. Herbs like brahmi in Ayurveda and schisandra in TCM are used to calm the mind and balance emotions during periods of heightened stress, especially around the Full Moon.

Western Research on Lunar Influence:

Studies published in Transcultural Psychiatry found an increase in psychiatric visits and heightened emotional crises during the Full Moon. Researchers theorized that the moon's bright light and gravitational forces amplify existing emotional conditions, making people more susceptible to anxiety, agitation, and even mania. While these effects may not be universal, the evidence supports the notion that lunar cycles influence emotional regulation.

Case Study: Emotional Healing Through Lunar Rituals

Sarah, who struggled with anxiety and emotional overwhelm, began incorporating Full Moon rituals into her wellness practice. Each Full Moon, she performed a releasing ceremony, writing down her burdens and burning the paper under the moon's light. Complementing this with calming herbal teas like chamomile and lavender during the Waning Moon, Sarah noticed significant improvements in her emotional health, demonstrating the healing potential of aligning self-care with lunar cycles.

Holistic Practices: Healing with the Moon's Phases

The moon's energy can enhance a variety of holistic healing practices, including herbal medicine, acupuncture, Reiki, and aromatherapy. Each lunar phase offers an opportunity to engage in practices that align with its energy.

Ayurveda and TCM Practices by Lunar Phase

New Moon: Ayurvedic Cleansing and Grounding

In Ayurveda, the New Moon is the perfect time for a gentle detox, grounding, and rebalancing. Use herbs like triphala to cleanse the digestive system and ashwagandha to ground the body's energy. Gentle yoga or meditation practices like Chandra Namaskar (moon salutation) help align the mind with the moon's quiet energy.

Waxing Moon: TCM for Energy and Growth

The Waxing Moon represents yang energy, a time for expansion and growth. TCM practitioners often recommend acupuncture sessions to stimulate energy flow during this phase. Use herbs like ginseng and schisandra to boost vitality and support emotional resilience.

Full Moon: Emotional Release with Reiki and Aromatherapy

The Full Moon, a time of heightened emotions, is ideal for Reiki sessions focused on releasing emotional blockages. Incorporating essential oils like frankincense and jasmine into Reiki or meditation practices enhances emotional clarity.

Waning Moon: TCM and Ayurvedic Reflection and Release

The Waning Moon is a time to release tension, cleanse the body, and prepare for renewal. TCM recommends soothing herbs like lotus seed or jujube for calming the mind and promoting deep rest. In Ayurveda, brahmi tea can be used to calm mental chatter and promote emotional release.

Herbal Medicine and the Moon

New Moon Herbs: Use grounding and cleansing herbs such as sage, chamomile, and burdock root to clear away stagnant energy and prepare for new beginnings.

Waxing Moon Herbs: Energizing herbs like rosemary, peppermint, and ginseng are ideal for supporting growth and action.

Full Moon Herbs: Mugwort, lavender, and jasmine are perfect for reflection and emotional clarity.

Waning Moon Herbs: Calming and purifying herbs such as lemon balm, skullcap, and valerian root help release emotional burdens.

Integrating Science, Spirit, and Holistic Healing

The moon offers us a pathway to balance and holistic healing. By integrating scientific understanding with ancient practices from Ayurveda, TCM, and Western holistic medicine, we can align our bodies, minds, and spirits with the natural world. Lunar phases provide a cyclical framework for mental and emotional well-being, and herbs, rituals, and alternative therapies deepen this connection.

Whether through science-backed research on sleep patterns and hormonal cycles or ancient practices of energy alignment, the moon remains a powerful guide for healing. By embracing its cycles, we can cultivate harmony within ourselves and our environment, fostering a deeper sense of peace, well-being, and connection to the cosmos. This holistic alignment allows us to approach wellness from multiple dimensions—physical, emotional, mental, and spiritual—honoring the balance between ancient wisdom and modern science.

Exploring Ancient Practices: Ayurveda and Traditional Chinese Medicine

The moon's influence on human health and spirituality has been recognized in ancient systems of healing like Ayurveda and Traditional Chinese Medicine (TCM) for thousands of years. These practices, deeply rooted in the natural world and its rhythms, provide valuable insight into how we can further our connection with the lunar cycle to enhance our holistic health.

Ayurveda: Balancing the Doshas with the Moon

In Ayurveda, one of the world's oldest healing systems, the moon is linked to the balance of the body's three doshas—Vata, Pitta, and Kapha. These doshas are energies that govern physical and mental processes and are influenced by the elements of air, fire, water, and earth.

- Vata (Air and Space): Vata, the dosha of movement, is influenced by the moon's waxing and waning. The moon's gravitational pull aligns with Vata's mobile nature, and this dosha is particularly active during the waxing phase. To balance Vata energy, practices like grounding foods, warm oil massages, and herbs such as ashwagandha and ginger are recommended, especially during the waxing and full moon.
- Pitta (Fire and Water): Pitta represents heat, metabolism, and transformation. The energy of the full moon can exacerbate Pitta imbalances, leading to increased emotions, irritability, or mental tension. Cooling herbs like coriander and mint, as well as calming practices like moon-gazing meditations, can help cool the fiery Pitta energy during this time.
- Kapha (Water and Earth): Kapha is associated with stability and structure, and its energy tends to dominate during the waning moon, a time

for slowing down and releasing. To keep Kapha energy in balance, stimulating practices like brisk walks and energizing herbal tonics with turmeric or black pepper are beneficial, especially as the moon's light fades.

Ayurveda teaches that by working with the moon's phases, we can bring harmony to our doshas, supporting both mental and physical health throughout the lunar cycle.

Traditional Chinese Medicine: Yin and Yang

In Traditional Chinese Medicine, the moon is closely tied to the balance of yin and yang—two complementary forces that regulate the body's internal energy. Yin represents rest, reflection, and cooling energy, while yang symbolizes action, heat, and vitality.

- Yin Phases (New and Waning Moon): These quieter phases of the moon are considered times for introspection, healing, and renewal. Yin herbs such as licorice root, peony, and rehmannia are used during these phases to nourish the body's fluids and support the emotional healing process. Practices like Tai Chi, Qigong, and acupuncture focused on balancing the body's meridians are ideal for this time, promoting inner calm and reflection.
- Yang Phases (Waxing and Full Moon): As the moon's energy builds, so does the body's yang energy. This is a time for taking action and focusing on physical and mental growth. Yang herbs, including ginseng, goji berry, and dang gui, can help strengthen the body's qi (life force), promoting vitality and movement. Exercises that encourage physical activity and circulation, like dynamic yoga or strength training, are

particularly effective during these phases.

By following the principles of TCM and incorporating herbal remedies and practices aligned with the moon's yin and yang phases, we can achieve a deeper balance between body, mind, and spirit.

Modern Western Medicine and the Moon's Influence

While the moon's impact on human health may not always be front and center in Western medicine, growing research and case studies demonstrate that the moon's cycles influence our biology in meaningful ways, especially in relation to sleep, hormonal health, and mental well-being.

The Science Behind Sleep and the Moon

As mentioned earlier, the moon's gravitational pull and light can disrupt sleep cycles, particularly during the Full Moon. While Western medicine often treats sleep disturbances with pharmaceutical interventions, there is increasing interest in natural remedies aligned with the lunar cycle. Practices such as sleep hygiene routines, mindfulness-based stress reduction, and herbal teas containing valerian and chamomile offer effective, non-invasive ways to combat the sleep disturbances that can arise during the moon's brighter phases.

Hormonal Health and Menstrual Cycles

Though Western medicine approaches hormone regulation through a clinical lens, with treatments often relying on synthetic hormones, an integrative approach looks at the body's natural rhythms. For example, as modern research suggests, the synchronization between menstrual cycles and lunar phases, while not definitive, points to the moon's subtle influence on hormonal health. Many women who adopt a holistic approach to managing menstrual health use the moon's phases to track fertility, emotional changes, and overall well-being.

Working with herbs like red raspberry leaf and evening primrose oil, alongside practices such as mindful eating, yoga, and cycle tracking apps, can offer Western medicine a natural complement to hormone regulation, helping to mitigate symptoms of PMS or menopause in a way that aligns with the lunar rhythm.

Expanding Your Lunar Healing Practice with Ancient and Modern Knowledge

As we combine the wisdom of ancient healing systems like Ayurveda and TCM with modern science, there are several ways to elevate your lunar healing practice to incorporate both spiritual and clinical approaches:

1. Create a Comprehensive Moon Phase Wellness Plan

- Map out your month based on the moon's phases, aligning each phase with specific practices. For example, you might schedule more intense physical workouts and goal-oriented projects during the waxing moon, while using the waning moon for emotional healing and reflection.

- Incorporate the recommended herbs, foods, and exercises from Ayurveda and TCM based on your personal needs and the doshic or yin/yang energies.

2. Integrate Modern Techniques with Ancient Wisdom

- If you're already practicing yoga or meditation, consider adding Ayurvedic herbs like brahmi or tulsi to your wellness routine for enhanced mental clarity during the New Moon. Similarly, incorporate TCM-inspired therapies such as acupuncture or gua sha during the Full Moon to release tension and emotional stagnation.
- Balance the spiritual with the practical by using modern sleep apps or meditation techniques to track how lunar phases affect your mental and physical well-being.

3. Journal and Reflect on Your Cyclical Wellness Journey

- Continue keeping a moon journal, but expand it to include any medical, emotional, or physical insights from both your spiritual and clinical practices. Pay attention to patterns in your energy, emotions, and health, and adjust your rituals or therapies accordingly.

By creating a bridge between ancient and modern practices, your lunar healing journey becomes more integrated, rooted in both tradition and evidence-based science.

Final Thoughts: Honoring the Union of Science, Spirit, and Holistic Healing

The moon's influence on our lives transcends time, culture, and geography. By acknowledging both ancient wisdom and modern scientific research, we open ourselves to a greater understanding of how the moon affects our bodies, minds, and spirits. Whether through Ayurveda's doshic balance, TCM's yin and yang principles, or the scientific studies linking lunar cycles to sleep and mood, the moon offers us a powerful framework for holistic healing.

As you continue your journey with the moon, may you embrace its cycles as a source of deep wisdom and healing, fostering harmony in both the visible and unseen aspects of your life. Let the integration of science and spirit serve as a guide for your own wellness, allowing you to move through life with more flow, grace, and understanding. The moon's cycles are not only a reflection of nature's rhythms but also a reflection of our own journey toward wholeness.

10

Aligning with the Moon and Nature's Rhythms for Holistic Wellness

The relationship between the moon and nature has been revered across cultures for centuries, a connection that mirrors the cycles of life, death, and rebirth. These lunar rhythms influence not just the tides of the ocean, but also the inner tides of our emotional, mental, and spiritual experiences. By tuning into the moon's phases, we unlock a deeper understanding of ourselves, how we move through the world, and how we can integrate the healing power of nature into our daily lives.

This chapter delves into how the moon's cycles offer a guide for harmonizing your wellness journey, providing you with practical and spiritual tools for a deeper connection to the world around you. We'll explore rituals, herbal practices, and self-care techniques to align your energy with the moon's phases, fostering greater mental, emotional, and physical well-being.

The Moon and Nature's Cycles: A Reflection of Life's Rhythms

The phases of the moon—New, Waxing, Full, and Waning—are a reflection of the larger rhythms found in nature. These cycles of growth, bloom, decay, and renewal align with the seasons and the natural processes of the Earth. Just as the Earth goes through cycles, so do we.

New Moon: The Quiet of Winter

The New Moon is akin to the energy of winter. It's a period of dormancy, stillness, and introspection. During this time, we are invited to go within and plant the seeds for future growth. It's the perfect moment for setting intentions, planning for the future, and embracing the quietude that allows for creativity to be born.

- Mindset: Reflective, introspective, focused on planning and new beginnings.
- Nature's Correspondence: Winter—trees are barren, animals hibernate, the earth is resting.

Waxing Moon: Springtime Awakening

As the moon begins to wax, increasing in light, the energy mirrors that of spring. This is a time for action, growth, and nurturing our intentions into reality. Just as spring brings budding flowers and new life, the Waxing Moon supports the active, outward expression of creativity and progress.

- Mindset: Energized, action-oriented, focused on building and manifesting.
- Nature's Correspondence: Spring—new growth, fresh beginnings, energy increases.

Full Moon: The Height of Summer

The Full Moon is the peak of the lunar cycle, representing fullness, abundance, and reflection. This phase aligns with the energy of summer, when life is at its most vibrant. It's a time to celebrate the progress you've made, reflect on the fruits of your labor, and express gratitude for the abundance around you.

- Mindset: Reflective, celebratory, focused on culmination and clarity.
- Nature's Correspondence: Summer—vibrant energy, fulfillment, fruition.

Waning Moon: The Release of Autumn

As the moon wanes and its light diminishes, it mirrors the energy of autumn, a time of release and transition. Just as autumn is a time for letting go—shedding leaves, preparing for rest—the Waning Moon encourages us to release what no longer serves us, creating space for renewal and inner peace.

- Mindset: Restorative, focused on release, letting go, and healing.
- Nature's Correspondence: Autumn—leaves fall, energy recedes, prepar-

ing for the rest of winter.

By embracing these natural cycles, we create harmony in our own lives, learning to move with the flow of the universe rather than against it. These rhythms teach us that there is a time for everything—growth, reflection, release, and rest.

Rituals for Deepening Connection to the Moon and Nature

Rituals are an opportunity to ground yourself in the rhythms of the moon and nature. They help us cultivate mindfulness and intention as we move through life's cycles, offering both spiritual and emotional support.

New Moon Ritual: Planting the Seeds of Intention

The New Moon is the perfect time to set goals and intentions for the upcoming lunar cycle. It's a phase of stillness, but also of potential—much like the dormant earth before spring.

Ritual: Write down your intentions for the next month. Bury them in soil or plant seeds as a symbolic gesture of your commitment to growth. Visualize these seeds sprouting and flourishing as the moon's light increases.

Incorporating Nature: If possible, spend time outdoors during the New Moon, even if it's just a few minutes sitting under the stars. This helps ground your intentions in the earth's energy. Work with grounding herbs like chamomile and sage to cleanse your space and create a fresh beginning.

Waxing Moon Ritual: Nurturing Your Growth

During the Waxing Moon, it's time to take action. This phase is about building on your intentions and nurturing the progress you've made.

Ritual: Go for a nature walk, collecting natural elements like stones, flowers, or leaves that symbolize growth to you. As you walk, reflect on the steps you've taken to move closer to your goals. Use these collected elements to create an altar or sacred space that serves as a reminder of your growth.

Incorporating Nature: Energize yourself with herbs like peppermint and rosemary. These herbs stimulate focus and motivation, making them perfect allies during the Waxing Moon.

Full Moon Ritual: Reflection and Celebration

The Full Moon is a time for celebration and gratitude. It's the peak of the lunar cycle, when we can reflect on what we've accomplished and release anything that no longer serves us.

Ritual: Stand under the Full Moon, taking deep breaths as you reflect on your journey over the past month. Write down things you're proud of, as well as anything you're ready to let go of. Burn the paper as a symbol of release.

Incorporating Nature: Lavender and mugwort are wonderful herbs for this phase, helping you relax and connect to your intuition. Use them in a bath or as a tea to support emotional clarity and healing.

Waning Moon Ritual: Letting Go

As the moon's light fades, it's time to turn inward and reflect on what needs to be released before the next cycle begins.

Ritual: Cleanse your space by smudging with sage or juniper. As you physically clear away clutter, focus on letting go of emotional or mental baggage. Meditate on what needs to be released and envision the moon drawing these things away.

Incorporating Nature: Create a calming tea with lemon balm, skullcap, and chamomile to soothe your mind and body as you prepare for the next cycle of growth.

Nature's Healing Power for Mental and Emotional Well-Being

One of the most profound ways to align with the moon is through nature itself. Studies show that spending time outdoors can reduce stress, lower anxiety, and improve mental health. Even small connections with nature, like taking a walk in a park or sitting by a body of water, can have a profound impact on emotional well-being.

- Grounding: Walking barefoot on the earth, also known as "earthing," can help balance your energy and reduce stress.
- Sunlight: Exposure to natural light, especially in the morning, supports healthy circadian rhythms and enhances mood.
- Greenery: Simply being in the presence of plants can improve air quality, reduce stress, and promote a sense of calm.

By incorporating time in nature into your lunar rituals, you amplify the healing energy of the moon and the Earth, fostering a deeper connection to the world around you and to yourself.

Final Thoughts: Embracing the Cycles of the Moon and Nature

In this chapter, we've explored the deep connection between the moon, nature, and our personal cycles of growth, rest, and renewal. By aligning your rituals, practices, and intentions with the lunar phases, you create a rhythm that mirrors the natural world, enhancing your mental, emotional, and spiritual well-being.

As you move forward, continue to explore how the moon's cycles influence your own energy, emotions, and growth. By embracing the rhythms of the moon and the Earth, you foster greater harmony within yourself, and in doing so, you open yourself to the endless possibilities of healing, transformation, and renewal.

Let these cycles be your guide as you move through life with grace, balance, and a deeper connection to both yourself and the universe.

11

Lunar-Inspired Meditation and Breathwork - Grounding the Spirit and Healing the Soul

Meditation and breathwork are powerful tools for self-discovery, healing, and spiritual growth. When integrated with the cycles of the moon, these practices become even more transformative, allowing you to align your inner rhythms with those of the Earth and sky. The moon's phases influence our emotional, mental, and spiritual states, and by tuning into these cycles through meditation and breathwork, we can cultivate greater balance, clarity, and healing.

In this chapter, we will explore various meditation and breathwork techniques designed to harness the unique energy of each lunar phase. Whether you seek grounding, release, or renewal, these practices will help you connect with the moon's cycles in a meaningful and profound way.

The Power of Meditation and Breathwork

Meditation and breathwork are age-old practices known for their ability to calm the mind, heal the spirit, and strengthen the connection between body and soul. Meditation centers your awareness, fostering clarity and emotional stability. Breathwork, on the other hand, uses the power of controlled breathing to regulate the nervous system, release emotional tension, and energize the body. When practiced together, they offer a holistic approach to wellness, allowing you to address both mental and physical imbalances.

By aligning these practices with the phases of the moon, you enhance their effectiveness, tapping into the lunar cycle's natural ebb and flow to create harmony within your mind and body. The moon has long been associated with intuition, emotional cycles, and spiritual insights. Through lunar-inspired meditation and breathwork, you connect with these ancient energies, promoting holistic wellness and spiritual growth.

Grounding Meditation for the New Moon

The New Moon represents a time of quiet potential, stillness, and new beginnings. This is the moment in the lunar cycle to turn inward, reflect on your desires, and plant the seeds for future growth. A grounding meditation during the New Moon helps you clear away distractions, anchor your energy, and cultivate focus as you set your intentions.

Meditation Instructions:

1. Find your space: Sit or lie down in a quiet place, ensuring you won't be disturbed. Close your eyes and take deep, slow breaths.
2. Visualize grounding energy: As you inhale, visualize roots extending from the base of your spine or feet, reaching deep into the earth. These roots provide stability, grounding you in the present moment.
3. Draw in the earth's energy: On each inhale, imagine drawing up nourishing energy from the earth, filling your body with peace and

stability. On each exhale, release any tension, fears, or worries into the earth, letting them dissolve.

4. Set intentions: Once grounded, focus on your intentions for the coming lunar cycle. What new projects, goals, or emotional shifts do you want to create? Visualize your intentions as seeds taking root in your energy field, ready to grow and thrive.

5. Close the meditation: Continue focusing on your breath and intentions for as long as feels comfortable. When ready, gently bring your awareness back to the room, taking this grounded energy with you as you move forward.

Waxing Moon Energizing Breathwork

As the moon waxes, building in light, it symbolizes growth, action, and the nurturing of intentions. This phase is ideal for building momentum and focusing on practical steps toward your goals. Breathwork during the Waxing Moon helps you harness this rising energy, providing motivation and vitality.

Breathwork Technique: Energizing Breath of Fire

1. Prepare your space: Sit comfortably with your spine straight, shoulders relaxed, and eyes closed.

2. Begin the breathwork: Start with a few deep breaths to center yourself. Then, begin breathing rapidly through your nose, with short, forceful exhales followed by quick inhales. Your diaphragm should move quickly and rhythmically, like a gentle pumping action.

3. Feel the energy build: As you continue this breathwork, feel the energy rising in your body. Visualize the Waxing Moon's light growing brighter with each breath, filling you with motivation, energy, and confidence.

4. Return to calm: After 1-2 minutes, return to slow, deep breathing. Feel the energy settle, and focus on the actions you need to take to nurture your intentions.

Full Moon Reflection Meditation

The Full Moon is a time of heightened energy, reflection, and release. As the moon reaches its peak, it illuminates all aspects of your life—your achievements, challenges, and emotional landscape. This is a time for celebrating successes and releasing anything that no longer serves your growth. Meditation during the Full Moon allows you to ground your energy, reflect on your journey, and let go of emotional burdens.

Meditation Instructions:

1. Get comfortable: Sit in a quiet space, close your eyes, and take several deep breaths to settle into the present moment.
2. Visualize the moon's light: As you inhale, imagine the light of the Full Moon shining down on you, filling your body with clarity and insight. Let this light bring awareness to any areas of your life that need reflection.
3. Release with each exhale: With each exhale, imagine releasing any emotions, thoughts, or attachments that are weighing you down. Visualize them dissolving in the moonlight, leaving you feeling lighter and more open.
4. Celebrate your progress: Take a moment to reflect on the accomplishments and growth you've experienced since the last Full Moon. Allow yourself to feel gratitude and pride in your journey.
5. Close the meditation: When you're ready, gently bring your awareness back to the present, carrying the clarity and release you've cultivated

with you.

Waning Moon Release Breathwork

As the moon begins to wane, its energy shifts toward reflection, release, and renewal. The Waning Moon invites us to let go of anything that no longer aligns with our highest good. Breathwork during this phase helps you release emotional and mental burdens, creating space for healing and renewal in the next lunar cycle.

Breathwork Technique: Slow Exhale Release

1. Prepare for release: Find a comfortable seated position. Begin with a few deep breaths to center your energy.
2. Breathe in deeply: Inhale slowly through your nose for a count of four. Hold the breath for a count of four, allowing the tension in your body to surface.
3. Exhale slowly: Exhale gently through your mouth for a count of eight. As you exhale, visualize releasing stress, negative thoughts, or emotional burdens. Feel them leave your body with each breath.
4. Repeat: Continue this breathwork for 5–10 minutes, allowing yourself to relax more deeply with each exhale. With each release, imagine yourself shedding layers of emotional and mental clutter, creating space for renewal.

Meditation and Breathwork for Mental Health and Healing

Meditation and breathwork offer potent benefits for mental and emotional health, especially when practiced in alignment with the moon's phases. Meditation provides a sanctuary from the busyness of life, helping you connect to your inner self and reduce anxiety, while breathwork regulates your nervous system, promoting calm and emotional balance.

- Meditation calms the mind, offering a sense of clarity, focus, and emotional resilience.
- Breathwork supports the body's natural ability to regulate emotions, releasing tension and helping you process stress.

By incorporating these practices into your life, especially in alignment with the lunar cycle, you create a cyclical pattern of healing and self-care. Grounding meditation during the New Moon helps you set intentions, energizing breathwork during the Waxing Moon builds momentum, reflective meditation during the Full Moon aids in emotional release, and release breathwork during the Waning Moon supports emotional renewal.

Recap of Lunar Meditation and Breathwork Practices

Each phase of the moon provides a unique opportunity for meditation and breathwork to enhance your holistic wellness:

- New Moon: Grounding meditation for intention-setting and stability.
- Waxing Moon: Energizing breathwork to build momentum and motiva-

tion.
- Full Moon: Reflection meditation to release emotional burdens and embrace clarity.
- Waning Moon: Slow exhale breathwork to let go of stress and emotional clutter.

By aligning these practices with the moon's phases, you deepen your connection to both your inner self and the natural world, fostering a greater sense of balance, peace, and emotional healing. These simple yet powerful tools will support your journey through each lunar cycle, helping you flow with the rhythms of the moon and your own evolving energy.

12

Herbal Crafting - Creating Healing Tools with Nature's Energy

Herbal crafting is a profound way to engage with the natural world, allowing you to create remedies that support your physical, emotional, and spiritual well-being. By crafting teas, balms, oils, and tinctures, you can harness the healing energy of plants, infuse them with your intentions, and align them with the lunar cycles to amplify their effects. This process not only provides you with potent tools for healing but also deepens your connection to the earth and its rhythms.

In this chapter, we will dive into the art of herbal crafting, exploring detailed techniques for creating healing teas, balms, infused oils, and tinctures. By pairing each craft with the corresponding lunar phase, you'll learn how to maximize the power of both the plants and the moon's energy to create effective and meaningful remedies.

The Healing Power of Herbal Teas: Nourishment from the Inside Out

Herbal teas are a simple yet powerful way to absorb the healing benefits of plants. By steeping herbs in hot water, you unlock their medicinal properties, which are easily absorbed by the body to nourish and balance you from the inside out. Teas can address a variety of health needs—whether it's mental clarity, emotional healing, or physical well-being.

Lunar Phase Pairing:

Herbal teas can be made to match any lunar phase, depending on your intention. For example, a tea created during the New Moon may focus on clarity and intention-setting, while a tea for the Waning Moon can aid in release and relaxation.

Clarity Tea for the New Moon

This blend is perfect for the New Moon phase when you are setting intentions and looking for mental clarity.

Ingredients:

- 1 tsp dried nettle
- 1 tsp dried peppermint
- 1 tsp dried rosemary

Instructions:

1. Boil a cup of water and add the herbs.
2. Let steep for 10-15 minutes to allow the full potency of the herbs to be extracted into the water.
3. As you drink, focus on clearing your mind and setting your intentions for the month ahead.

Tip: Add a touch of honey for extra grounding and sweetness.

Herbal Infused Oils: Healing for the Skin and Spirit

Herbal-infused oils are another versatile craft that offers both physical and spiritual benefits. By infusing herbs in a carrier oil, you extract the medicinal compounds of the plants, which can then be applied to the skin for nourishment, healing, and ritual anointing.

Lunar Phase Pairing:
Infused oils can be created during the Waxing Moon to promote growth and abundance or the Waning Moon for release and protection. Infusions during the Full Moon are particularly powerful for drawing out the full energy of the herbs for manifestation and healing.

Energizing Infused Oil for the Waxing Moon

This oil blend uses stimulating herbs to promote mental focus and energy, making it perfect for the Waxing Moon when growth and action are in focus.

Ingredients:

- 1 cup sunflower oil (or another carrier oil)
- 2 tbsp dried rosemary
- 1 tbsp dried peppermint
- 1 tbsp dried ginseng root

Instructions:

1. Place the dried herbs in a glass jar and pour the oil over them, ensuring the herbs are fully submerged.
2. Seal the jar tightly and leave it in a warm, sunny place for 2-3 weeks, shaking gently each day.
3. After the infusion period, strain the oil using a cheesecloth.
4. Store the oil in a dark glass bottle in a cool place.
5. Use the oil for self-massage, in a bath, or to anoint your body during rituals.

Tip: To energize your morning routine, rub a small amount on your temples for focus and mental clarity.

Herbal Balms: Protection, Soothing, and Nourishment

Herbal balms are practical and effective for skin care, muscle aches, and ritual protection. By combining healing herbs with a base of beeswax and oils, you create a nourishing salve that can protect your skin and support emotional healing.

Lunar Phase Pairing:
Craft your balms during the Waning Moon for protection and grounding, or

during the Full Moon when the energy of release and healing is at its peak.

Protection Balm for the Waning Moon

This balm harnesses the protective qualities of herbs like mugwort and rosemary, providing both physical and energetic shielding.

Ingredients:

- 1/2 cup coconut oil
- 1/4 cup beeswax
- 2 tbsp dried mugwort
- 2 tbsp dried rosemary
- 1 tbsp dried sage
- 10 drops lavender essential oil (optional)

Instructions:

1. Melt the coconut oil and beeswax in a double boiler.
2. Remove from heat and stir in the dried herbs. Let the mixture infuse for 30 minutes.
3. Strain the herbs from the oil and reheat the infused oil in the double boiler.
4. Pour the mixture into small tins or jars and let cool until solid.
5. Use during rituals by anointing your pulse points or rubbing a small amount on your feet to stay grounded.

Tip: Carry this balm with you for grounding and protection throughout the day.

Herbal Tinctures: Potent and Powerful Healing

Tinctures are highly concentrated herbal remedies that offer profound healing with just a few drops. By extracting the active ingredients of herbs in alcohol or vinegar, tinctures deliver fast, potent results.

Lunar Phase Pairing:
  Tinctures benefit greatly from being made during the Full Moon when the energy is ripe for manifestation and healing, but they can be created during any lunar phase depending on the intention.

Healing Tincture for Emotional Release during the Full Moon

This tincture supports emotional healing and mental balance, using herbs that calm the nervous system and promote deep emotional release.

Ingredients:

- 1 cup vodka (or Apple Cider Vinegar)
- 1 tbsp dried skullcap
- 1 tbsp dried valerian root
- 1 tbsp dried passionflower

Instructions:

1. Place the dried herbs in a glass jar and cover with vodka.
2. Seal the jar tightly and store it in a cool, dark place for 4-6 weeks, shaking gently each day.
3. After 4-6 weeks, strain the herbs and pour the tincture into dark glass dropper bottles.
4. Take 1-2 drops as needed for emotional support.

Tip: Use this tincture during Full Moon meditations to support emotional balance and release.

Lunar Herbal Crafting for Mental Health

Herbal crafting isn't just about physical healing—it's also a deeply meditative and emotional practice. When done with intention, herbal remedies can become allies in your mental health journey, providing tools for grounding, clarity, emotional release, and renewal.

For example, crafting a Protection Balm during the Waning Moon helps ground your energy during times of emotional turmoil. Or, you might create a Healing Tincture during the Full Moon to help you process deep emotions.

By tuning into the cycles of the moon and engaging in mindful crafting, you bring yourself into a state of flow with nature, where healing is both intentional and holistic.

Recap of Herbal Crafting Techniques

In this chapter, we've explored several methods of herbal crafting, from teas to tinctures, each aligned with the lunar phases to maximize their healing potential. These herbal remedies not only support your physical health but also nurture your emotional and spiritual well-being.

- Teas: Gentle yet powerful, teas can be created to support everything from mental clarity to emotional release.
- Infused Oils: Versatile and potent, these oils can be used for physical healing or spiritual anointing.
- Balms: Herbal balms provide a protective, grounding layer for both body and spirit.
- Tinctures: Potent and concentrated, tinctures offer fast and effective healing for deep emotional and physical imbalances.

By embracing the art of herbal crafting and working in harmony with the lunar phases, you can create healing tools that enhance your wellness journey and connect you more deeply with the rhythms of nature and the moon.

13

Sacred Lunar Rituals and Herbal Remedies - Enhancing Your Healing Journey

These rituals are not simply about performing an act; they are an invitation to connect deeply with the moon, with nature, and with yourself. Each practice has evolved through my personal journey as I incorporated them into my life to cope with struggles and heal. My hope is that they bring you the same comfort, clarity, and empowerment as they have brought me.

Lunar Flame Release Ritual

This ritual focuses on letting go of what no longer serves you, using the transformative power of fire under the full moon.

Materials:

- A fire-safe bowl or cauldron
- A small piece of paper and pen
- Matches or a lighter

- Sage or incense (optional, for cleansing)

Instructions:

1. Prepare Your Space: Find a quiet, outdoor space where you can see the full moon. Light sage or incense to cleanse the area and yourself.
2. Set Your Intention: Reflect on what emotional, physical, or spiritual burdens you want to release. Write them down on a piece of paper.
3. Call Upon Lunar Energy: Close your eyes and take several deep breaths, visualizing the full moon's light enveloping you. Imagine its energy filling you with the power to release and transform.
4. Burn the Paper: Safely light the paper, saying aloud or in your mind, "I release all that no longer serves me. I am open to new growth and transformation."
5. Let Go: Allow the paper to burn fully, visualizing your burdens disintegrating with the flames. Sit with the moonlight for a few moments, feeling lighter and freer.

Moon-Infused Herbal Elixir

This ritual is designed to infuse your herbal preparations with the powerful energy of the moon.

Materials:

- A jar of clean water
- Fresh or dried herbs of your choice (e.g., lavender, rosemary, or

chamomile)
- A clear glass container with a lid

Instructions:

1. Prepare Your Herbal Blend: Choose herbs that align with your intention for the water (e.g., lavender for peace, rosemary for protection, chamomile for healing). Place the herbs in a jar of clean water.
2. Place Under the Full Moon: Set your jar outside where it can soak up the full moon's energy overnight.
3. Invoke the Moon's Power: As you place the jar down, say, "By the light of the moon, may these herbs be charged with healing, love, and strength."
4. Harvest the Water: In the morning, retrieve the jar and strain out the herbs. The moon-infused water can now be used in bath rituals, for anointing tools, or in other herbal creations like teas or body sprays.

Cinnamon Prosperity Manifestation

This ritual uses the fiery energy of cinnamon to attract abundance and success.

Materials:

- Ground cinnamon
- A small bowl
- A green candle (symbolizing wealth and prosperity)

Instructions:

1. Prepare Your Candle: Before the ritual, cleanse the candle by rubbing it down with a little oil (e.g., olive oil). Roll it in the cinnamon, coating it lightly.
2. Set Your Intention: Sit quietly and think about the specific prosperity or abundance you want to attract. Hold the candle in your hands and visualize yourself achieving your desires.
3. Light the Candle: As you light the green candle, say aloud, "With the power of cinnamon, I manifest prosperity and abundance into my life."
4. Sprinkle Cinnamon: Stand at your front door, facing inside your home. Take a pinch of cinnamon and blow it through the door while saying, "As this cinnamon blows, abundance flows."
5. Let the Candle Burn: Let the candle burn down completely (or at least for a few hours). Visualize prosperity flowing into your life.

Incense of Release Ritual

This ritual helps to symbolically release emotional or spiritual baggage using the purifying qualities of incense.

Materials:

- Incense sticks or cones (sandalwood, frankincense, or lavender)
- A fireproof dish or incense holder
- A journal and pen

Instructions:

1. Create a Sacred Space: Light your incense and let the smoke fill your space. Allow the scent to center and ground you.
2. Reflect on What You Wish to Release: With your journal, write down any lingering emotions, toxic relationships, or unhealthy habits you wish to let go of.
3. Offer Your Release to the Smoke: Hold the paper where you've written your thoughts, passing it through the incense smoke. Visualize the smoke carrying these thoughts away.
4. Burn or Bury the Paper: Tear up the paper and either burn it safely or bury it outside under the moon. As you do so, say, "I release what no longer serves me. I make space for new growth and healing."
5. Conclude with Gratitude: Close the ritual by thanking the moon, the incense, and the elements for their support. Take a few deep breaths, feeling the release and sense of renewal.

Lavender Dream Sachet for Sleep and Intuition

This ritual is perfect for enhancing intuitive dreams and promoting restful sleep, especially during the Full Moon or Waning Moon.

Materials:

- Dried lavender flowers
- Dried mugwort (optional, for intuitive dreaming)
- A small cloth pouch
- A piece of amethyst or clear quartz

Instructions:

1. Create the Sachet: Place the dried lavender and mugwort in a small cloth pouch. Add the crystal to amplify the sachet's energy.
2. Set Your Intention: Hold the sachet in your hands and set the intention for restful sleep and intuitive dreams. Say, "May this sachet bring peace to my sleep and insight to my dreams."
3. Place Under Your Pillow: Keep the sachet under your pillow while you sleep, allowing the herbs and crystal to work their magic.
4. Reflect on Dreams: In the morning, take a few moments to reflect on any dreams or insights you received. Keep a journal by your bedside to write down any messages.

Rose and Chamomile Heart-Healing Bath

This ritual is perfect for nurturing self-love and emotional healing, especially during the Waning Moon or Full Moon.

Materials:

- Dried rose petals
- Dried chamomile flowers
- Epsom salts
- A few drops of rose essential oil

Instructions:

1. Prepare the Bath: Fill your bathtub with warm water and add the dried rose petals, chamomile flowers, and Epsom salts. Add a few drops of rose essential oil for emotional healing.
2. Set Your Intention: As the bath fills, take a moment to set your intention for healing and self-love. Say, "I am open to love and healing. I release all emotional pain and invite peace into my heart."
3. Soak in the Bath: Relax in the bath for at least 20 minutes, allowing the herbs and salts to soothe your body and spirit.
4. Reflect: After your bath, spend a few moments journaling or meditating on any emotions or insights that came up during the ritual.

Prosperity Herbal Sachet

This simple sachet is designed to attract abundance and prosperity into your life, using the energy of the Waxing Moon.

Materials:

- Dried basil (for abundance)
- Dried cinnamon (for success)
- A small green cloth pouch
- A piece of citrine or green aventurine

Instructions:

1. Create the Sachet: Place the dried herbs and crystal in a small green cloth pouch.

2. Set Your Intention: Hold the sachet in your hands and set your intention for prosperity and success. Say, "I attract abundance and prosperity into my life with ease and grace."
3. Keep the Sachet in Your Space: Place the sachet on your altar, in your wallet, or in a prominent area where you are working on financial goals.
4. Reinforce the Intention: Repeat the affirmation whenever you hold the sachet or whenever you feel the need to attract abundance.

With these sacred practices, I hope you find the peace, strength, and guidance that the moon has always offered me on my journey. Each ritual is an opportunity to connect with the moon, with nature, and with yourself— helping you align your energy, release what no longer serves you, and invite healing and abundance into your life. Let these practices serve as reminders that you are supported, loved, and capable of manifesting your highest potential.

14

Moon Rituals for Specific Life Events - Honoring Transitions and Life's Milestones

Life is filled with moments of transition, whether they be joyous beginnings, challenging losses, or moments of deep personal transformation. The moon, with its ever-shifting phases, serves as a powerful mirror for these life events. By aligning specific rituals with key lunar phases, we can create sacred practices that honor and support us through each milestone in our lives. These rituals not only offer healing but also provide a sense of grounding and connection to the natural cycles of the universe.

New Beginnings Ritual: Welcoming New Chapters

Lunar Phase: New Moon

Whether you're embarking on a new career, moving into a new home, starting a relationship, or transitioning into parenthood, the New Moon provides fertile ground for planting the seeds of intention. It represents a blank slate, a fresh start, and a chance to align your energy with the possibilities ahead.

Materials:

- A small plant or seedling
- A clean notebook or journal
- A candle (white or green for new growth)
- Essential oil (such as rosemary or peppermint for clarity)

Instructions:

1. Set the Space: Find a quiet place where you feel connected to the earth. Light your candle to symbolize the beginning of a new chapter. Anoint your wrists or third eye with a few drops of essential oil to clear your mind.
2. Reflect and Set Intentions: Take a few deep breaths, allowing yourself to settle into the moment. In your journal, write down your hopes and intentions for this new beginning. What do you want to cultivate or manifest? Be specific and let your heart guide you.
3. Plant Your Seedling: Gently plant the seedling in a pot or garden. As you cover the roots with soil, visualize your intentions taking root in the physical world. Speak them aloud if you feel called to do so.
4. Nurture and Grow: Keep the plant in a spot where you will see it regularly. As it grows, use it as a reminder of your new beginnings and the energy you are cultivating. Tend to it with care, just as you tend to your intentions.

Grief and Loss Ritual: Finding Peace in Letting Go

Lunar Phase: Waning Moon or New Moon

Grief and loss are universal experiences, yet they can feel deeply isolating. During times of loss—whether it be the end of a relationship, the death of a loved one, or the closing of a significant chapter—the Waning Moon offers a supportive time for release, surrender, and healing. This ritual is designed to gently guide you through the process of letting go, while still holding space for healing and remembrance.

Materials:

- A photograph or memento related to the loss
- A bowl of water (symbolizing the flow of emotions)
- A candle (black or dark blue for release)
- Lavender essential oil for comfort and peace

Instructions:

1. Create a Safe Space: Light the candle and place the bowl of water in front of you. Add a few drops of lavender essential oil to the water. Sit quietly, taking deep breaths, and allow your emotions to surface. There is no need to rush this process—grief takes time.
2. Reflect on the Loss: Hold the memento or photograph in your hands, and gently reflect on what this loss means to you. Acknowledge the emotions that come up, whether they be sadness, anger, or confusion.
3. Release through Water: When you're ready, dip your fingers into the

bowl of water. As you do so, speak aloud what you are ready to release: "I release this pain. I release this attachment. I allow healing to flow through me." Visualize your pain flowing into the water, being cleansed and transformed.

4. Let Go: Finally, pour the water onto the earth (either outside or into a potted plant), symbolizing the release of your grief back into nature. Extinguish the candle, giving thanks for the healing power of the moon and the cycle of life.

Celebration and Gratitude Ritual: Honoring Milestones

Lunar Phase: Full Moon

Milestones are a time for celebration, reflection, and gratitude. Whether you're celebrating a personal achievement, an anniversary, or simply want to express gratitude for the abundance in your life, the Full Moon offers the perfect energy for amplifying joy and giving thanks.

Materials:

- A bouquet of fresh flowers (symbolizing growth and beauty)
- A journal or piece of paper
- A candle (gold or yellow for joy)
- Rose or jasmine essential oil for self-love and beauty

Instructions:

1. Prepare for Celebration: Choose a special space where you can feel the energy of the Full Moon. Light your candle and surround yourself with the flowers. Anoint your wrists with rose or jasmine essential oil to invite a sense of love and celebration.

2. Express Gratitude: Take your journal and write down all the things you are grateful for—big or small. Be specific, and focus on the feelings of joy, abundance, and pride in your heart. If you're celebrating a specific milestone, reflect on the journey that led you here.

3. Create a Flower Offering: When you're ready, gather the petals from your bouquet and release them into nature—whether in a river, lake, or a garden—symbolizing the return of your gratitude to the earth. As you do so, say, "I honor this moment and give thanks for the blessings in my life. I open myself to continued growth and abundance."

4. Celebrate: Take a moment to bask in the energy of the Full Moon and the feelings of joy and accomplishment. Feel the universe supporting your growth and success.

Transformation Ritual: Embracing Change

Lunar Phase: Waxing Moon or Full Moon

Change is often uncomfortable, but it's also where deep growth occurs. Whether you're experiencing an internal transformation or an external life shift, the Waxing Moon is an ideal time to welcome change with courage and trust.

Materials:

- A feather (representing freedom and lightness)
- A candle (purple for transformation)
- Sage or incense for cleansing
- A small mirror for reflection

Instructions:

1. Prepare the Space: Light your candle and cleanse the space with sage or incense. Place the feather and mirror in front of you, inviting a sense of clarity and peace into your heart.
2. Visualize the Change: Close your eyes and bring to mind the change you're currently experiencing. Allow yourself to feel the emotions that come with this shift, whether they're fear, excitement, or uncertainty.
3. Reflect in the Mirror: Take the mirror and look into it, seeing yourself not as you are now, but as the person you are becoming. Visualize this transformation, and speak aloud any affirmations that reflect your courage and trust: "I am evolving. I trust this process of growth. I embrace the person I am becoming."
4. Release with the Feather: Take the feather and lightly wave it around your body, symbolizing the lightness of release and the freedom that comes with change. As you do, imagine any resistance to change leaving your body, replaced by a sense of peace and acceptance.

15

Self-Care Rituals for Busy Lives - Nurturing Your Mind, Body, and Spirit in Small, Powerful Moments

In today's fast-paced world, finding time for self-care can often feel like a luxury. However, the truth is that caring for your mind, body, and spirit is essential to maintaining balance and wellness—especially when life is busy. The good news is that self-care doesn't need to take hours or require elaborate rituals. Even small, intentional moments can create lasting effects on your overall well-being.

In this chapter, we'll explore simple, yet powerful, self-care practices that fit seamlessly into your busy lifestyle. These rituals are designed to help you ground, restore, and nurture yourself, no matter how hectic your schedule may be. By weaving mindfulness and intention into your daily routine, you'll discover that self-care can be both accessible and transformative.

Morning Rituals to Set the Tone for Your Day

The way you start your morning sets the tone for the rest of your day. Even if you're pressed for time, dedicating just a few minutes to self-care in the morning can help you approach your day with clarity, focus, and calm.

Mindful Morning Breathing (2-5 Minutes)

1. Before reaching for your phone or diving into your to-do list, take a few moments for mindful breathing. Sit up in bed or find a comfortable seated position, close your eyes, and place your hands over your heart. Take a deep inhale through your nose, filling your lungs completely, and then exhale slowly through your mouth.

2. Repeat this cycle of deep breathing for 2-5 minutes, focusing on the sensation of your breath and allowing any tension or stress to melt away. As you breathe, set an intention for how you want to approach your day—whether it's with focus, ease, or gratitude.

Herbal Tea for Grounding and Energy (5-10 Minutes)

1. If you're a tea drinker, use the act of preparing your morning tea as a grounding ritual. Choose an herbal blend that supports energy and clarity, such as peppermint or rosemary, and take a moment to inhale the aroma of the herbs as they steep.

2. As you sip your tea, practice mindfulness by focusing on the warmth of the cup in your hands, the taste of the tea on your tongue, and the way the herbs make you feel. This simple act of presence can help you center yourself before the day's demands take hold.

Quick Movement for Energy (5-10 Minutes)

1. If your mornings feel rushed, a few minutes of mindful movement can make a big difference in how you feel. Whether it's a few gentle stretches, a quick yoga flow, or a brisk walk around your home, moving your body helps increase circulation, release tension, and boost energy.

2. Focus on the connection between your breath and your body as you move, allowing this time to be a moment of physical and mental release. Even 5 minutes of movement can leave you feeling refreshed and ready for the day ahead.

Midday Rituals for Recalibrating and Recharging

As the day progresses, it's common to experience a dip in energy, focus, or mood. By incorporating small self-care rituals into your midday routine, you can recalibrate your energy and maintain a sense of balance throughout the day.

Grounding Visualization (3-5 Minutes)

1. When you're feeling overwhelmed or scattered, a quick grounding visualization can help you recenter and refocus. Close your eyes and take a few deep breaths. As you inhale, imagine roots growing from the soles of your feet and extending deep into the earth. Feel these roots anchoring you, providing stability and strength.

2. As you exhale, imagine any stress, tension, or distractions leaving your body and being absorbed by the earth. Continue this visualization for 3-5 minutes, allowing yourself to feel grounded, calm, and supported.

Hydration and Herbal Support (5 Minutes)

1. Hydration is one of the simplest yet most effective forms of self-care. Throughout the day, stay mindful of your body's need for water. For an added layer of nourishment, infuse your water with herbs like mint or lemon balm, which support mental clarity and emotional balance.
2. If you prefer tea, opt for a mid-afternoon cup of green tea or an herbal blend with energizing properties, such as ginseng or lemongrass. As you drink, take a moment to check in with yourself—how are you feeling physically, mentally, and emotionally?

Mindful Stretching (5-10 Minutes)

1. Whether you're at a desk, running errands, or managing a household, tension can build up in your muscles, particularly in the neck, shoulders, and back. Take a few minutes midday to release that tension with mindful stretching.
2. Focus on slow, intentional movements, gently stretching your neck, shoulders, arms, and legs. As you stretch, breathe deeply, and allow your body to soften and release any tightness. This practice not only reduces physical discomfort but also helps clear mental fog and restore focus.

Evening Rituals for Winding Down and Relaxation

Incorporating self-care into your evening routine is essential for releasing the stress of the day and preparing your mind and body for restful sleep. These rituals help you transition from the demands of the day into a state of calm and relaxation.

Candlelight Meditation (5-10 Minutes)

1. At the end of a long day, light a candle and use it as the focal point for a short meditation. Sit comfortably in a quiet space, with the candle in front of you. As you gaze softly at the flame, take slow, deep breaths, allowing the warmth and glow of the candle to calm your mind.

2. As you meditate, visualize any stress or tension dissolving in the light of the flame. Focus on the present moment and allow yourself to let go of any lingering thoughts or worries from the day.

Herbal Bath or Foot Soak (15-20 Minutes)

1. Water has a natural ability to cleanse and heal both the body and the spirit. If you have time for a bath, create a relaxing ritual by adding calming herbs such as lavender, chamomile, or rose petals to the water. If a full bath isn't possible, a simple foot soak can have the same grounding and relaxing effect.

2. As you soak, close your eyes and focus on the sensation of the water and the calming aroma of the herbs. Use this time to reflect on the day, acknowledging what you accomplished and gently letting go of anything that didn't go as planned.

Gratitude Journal (5 Minutes)

1. Before bed, take a few moments to reflect on your day and write down three things you're grateful for. This practice shifts your focus away from stress or negativity and reminds you of the positive moments, however small, that each day holds.

2. Gratitude journaling helps to reframe your perspective, fostering a sense

of contentment and peace as you prepare for rest. It also creates a positive mindset that carries over into the following day.

Self-Care and the Lunar Phases

Just as the moon moves through phases, our energy and needs change throughout the month. Aligning your self-care rituals with the lunar cycle allows you to work with the natural ebb and flow of your energy, ensuring that your self-care practices support you in a holistic way.

New Moon

A time for setting intentions, planting seeds, and focusing on new beginnings. Practice self-care by journaling your goals, meditating on your intentions, or engaging in a cleansing ritual like smudging or bathing.

Waxing Moon

As the moon grows in light, your energy begins to rise. This is a time for action, growth, and building momentum. Focus on self-care that energizes and motivates you, such as energizing breathwork, yoga, or invigorating herbal teas.

Full Moon

The Full Moon is a time of culmination, reflection, and release. Practice self-care by reflecting on what you've accomplished, celebrating your progress, and releasing what no longer serves you. Engage in rituals like journaling, releasing ceremonies, or soaking in a bath with herbs for emotional healing.

Waning Moon

As the moon's light begins to fade, your energy may naturally begin to slow down. This is a time for rest, introspection, and letting go. Focus on self-care practices that promote relaxation and renewal, such as restorative yoga, meditation, or herbal teas that calm and soothe.

Integrating Self-Care into Everyday Life

The key to consistent self-care is recognizing that it doesn't have to be time-consuming or complicated. By weaving small rituals into your day—whether it's a few minutes of mindful breathing in the morning, a quick stretch midday, or a gratitude practice before bed—you create a sustainable self-care routine that fits your life.

The more you practice self-care, the more you'll notice its benefits—reduced stress, increased clarity, better sleep, and a deeper sense of connection to yourself. Even in the busiest of seasons, these simple rituals remind you to pause, breathe, and prioritize your well-being.

Remember, self-care isn't selfish—it's essential. By nurturing yourself, you're better equipped to show up fully for the people and responsibilities in your life, and you'll feel more grounded, energized, and balanced in the process.

16

Holistic Wellness Beyond the Moon - Expanding Your Practice to Connect with Nature and Self

While the moon provides a powerful guide for personal growth, healing, and transformation, there are many other natural cycles, practices, and elements that can deepen your holistic wellness journey. True wellness encompasses all aspects of life—the mind, body, spirit, and the natural world around us. In this chapter, we'll explore how to take your lunar practice further by integrating elements of nature, mindfulness, and traditional holistic practices into your daily routine.

Aligning with the Seasons

Just as the moon moves through its phases, the seasons represent larger cycles of change and transformation. Tuning into the energy of each season can bring balance and flow into your life, allowing you to work with the natural rhythms of the earth to support your wellness journey.

Spring (Renewal and Growth)

- Spring is a time of rebirth and fresh beginnings. As nature comes to life, it invites us to plant seeds of intention, both literally and metaphorically. Use this time to focus on new projects, personal growth, and clearing away the stagnation of winter.
- Practice: Engage in a spring-cleaning ritual—both in your home and in your energy field. Smudge your space with sage or rosemary to clear away old energy, and perform a grounding meditation in nature to align with the new growth around you.

Summer (Abundance and Expansion)

- The summer season is one of fullness, abundance, and outward expression. It's a time to enjoy the fruits of your labor and celebrate the joy in your life. This is also a powerful time for manifestation, as the energy is high and vibrant.
- Practice: Spend time outdoors, soaking up the sun's energy. Create a gratitude journal to celebrate your achievements, and incorporate solar herbs like St. John's Wort and calendula into your rituals for vitality and protection.

Autumn (Harvest and Release)

- Autumn marks a time of harvesting, reflection, and letting go. As the leaves fall, we are reminded of the beauty in release and the necessity of surrendering what no longer serves us.
- Practice: Perform a gratitude harvest ritual by writing down everything you've achieved and gathered throughout the year. Reflect on what you are ready to release and make space for renewal. Work with herbs like cinnamon and ginger for grounding warmth and energy.

Winter (Rest and Reflection)

- Winter is a time of stillness, deep introspection, and rest. Just as nature retreats and regenerates, so too should we slow down and focus on inner healing and replenishment.
- Practice: Use this time for self-care, reflection, and restoration. Incorporate warming teas and baths into your routine, using herbs like chamomile and valerian for deep relaxation. Create a self-love ritual by setting intentions for healing and inner peace during this quiet season.

The Power of Mindfulness

Mindfulness is the practice of being fully present in the moment, without judgment or distraction. It is a foundational aspect of holistic wellness because it helps us to reconnect with our bodies, our emotions, and the world around us. Mindfulness can be integrated into every part of your life, from eating and walking to working and relaxing.

Simple Mindfulness Practices to Enhance Your Wellness:

- Mindful Breathing: Take a few moments throughout your day to pause and focus on your breath. Inhale deeply through your nose, feeling the air fill your lungs, and exhale slowly through your mouth. As you breathe, focus on the sensation of air moving through your body, and let go of any tension or distraction. This practice instantly brings you back to the present moment, calming the mind and grounding the spirit.
- Mindful Eating: Before you eat, take a moment to appreciate your food— its colors, textures, and aroma. As you eat, chew slowly and savor each

bite. Notice how your body feels as you nourish it, and practice gratitude for the meal in front of you. This practice not only improves digestion but also deepens your connection to the food that sustains you.

- Mindful Walking: Whether you're walking in nature or simply moving through your home, bring awareness to each step. Feel the ground beneath your feet, notice the rhythm of your body, and observe your surroundings with fresh eyes. Walking mindfully helps to release stress, increase focus, and bring a sense of calm to your day.

Traditional Healing Practices

In addition to working with the moon and natural cycles, integrating traditional healing practices from around the world can provide powerful support for your holistic wellness journey. These practices have been used for centuries to promote balance, healing, and spiritual growth.

Ayurveda:

- An ancient Indian system of medicine, Ayurveda focuses on balancing the body's doshas (vata, pitta, and kapha) to promote health and harmony. By understanding your unique constitution, you can tailor your diet, lifestyle, and self-care practices to align with your natural energy.
- Practice: Begin incorporating Ayurvedic principles into your life by determining your dosha and adjusting your daily habits to balance your energies. For example, if you are predominantly vata, focus on grounding routines, warming foods, and calming practices to stabilize your airy nature.

Traditional Chinese Medicine (TCM):

- TCM is based on the concept of balancing the body's qi (life force) through practices such as acupuncture, herbal medicine, and tai chi. This system works with the body's energy meridians to promote overall health and vitality.
- Practice: Start by learning basic TCM principles, such as the balance of yin and yang and how they influence your body and emotions. Incorporate practices like qi gong or acupressure into your wellness routine to balance your energy flow and support long-term health.

Reiki:

- Reiki is a Japanese energy healing practice that involves channeling universal life force energy through the hands to balance the body's energy centers (chakras). Reiki is a gentle yet powerful tool for reducing stress, promoting relaxation, and supporting emotional healing.
- Practice: If you are new to Reiki, consider receiving a session from a certified practitioner to experience its benefits firsthand. You can also explore self-Reiki techniques to ground and center your energy at home, especially during moments of emotional overwhelm or physical exhaustion.

Embracing Daily Rituals

Rituals don't have to be reserved for the New Moon or Full Moon. By creating small daily rituals, you can bring sacredness and intention to every part of your life. These daily practices help anchor you in the present and create a sense of rhythm, helping you stay connected to your goals and intentions.

Ideas for Daily Rituals:

- Morning Ritual: Start your day with a few moments of quiet reflection or meditation. Set an intention for how you want to show up in the world, and take a moment to visualize your day unfolding with ease and grace. You can also brew a cup of herbal tea, using the act of preparing and drinking your tea as a grounding practice to center your mind and body.
- Midday Check-In: Around midday, take a break from your tasks to check in with yourself. How are you feeling physically, emotionally, and mentally? If you're feeling off-balance, take a few deep breaths, stretch your body, or step outside for fresh air. This simple act of self-care can prevent stress from building up and help you maintain clarity and focus.
- Evening Wind-Down: As the day comes to a close, create a peaceful space for rest and reflection. You might light a candle, diffuse calming essential oils, or practice gentle stretching or yoga. Take time to journal or meditate, reflecting on the events of the day and releasing any tension or worry. This practice prepares your body and mind for restful sleep.

Honoring the Elements

The four elements—earth, air, fire, and water—are foundational to holistic wellness. By working with these elements, you can create rituals and practices that balance and align your energy with the natural world.

- Earth: The element of grounding, stability, and physicality. Work with earth energy through grounding practices like walking barefoot on the ground, gardening, or holding stones or crystals.
- Air: The element of intellect, clarity, and communication. Incorporate air

by practicing deep breathing, focusing on mental clarity, or working with herbs like peppermint and eucalyptus to stimulate the mind.

- Fire: The element of transformation, action, and passion. Light candles, work with cinnamon or ginger, or engage in physical exercise to activate fire energy in your life.
- Water: The element of emotions, intuition, and flow. Work with water through bathing rituals, spending time near lakes or rivers, and using herbs like chamomile and lemon balm to soothe and relax the emotions.

17

Personalizing Your Lunar Journey - Crafting a Unique and Intuitive Relationship with the Moon

As we've explored throughout this book, the moon's cycles offer a powerful framework for aligning our lives with the natural rhythms of the universe. But while the lunar phases provide structure and guidance, the true power of working with the moon lies in personalizing your experience and crafting a journey that feels authentic to you.

In this chapter, we'll dive deep into how you can create a customized lunar practice that speaks to your unique needs, goals, and intuitive wisdom. Whether you're drawn to specific moon phases, rituals, or healing practices, this chapter will guide you in building a relationship with the moon that is flexible, deeply personal, and aligned with your spirit.

Understanding Your Relationship with the Moon

Before you begin to personalize your lunar journey, it's important to reflect on your current relationship with the moon and how it resonates with you. The moon's energy affects each of us differently, and by paying attention to how you respond to its phases, you can begin to uncover patterns in your emotional, mental, and physical state.

Questions for Reflection:

- During which lunar phases do you feel most energized? When do you feel the need to slow down and reflect?
- Are there specific rituals, meditations, or healing practices that resonate with you more during certain moon phases?
- How do your goals, intentions, or emotions shift as the moon waxes and wanes? Do you notice patterns in your productivity, creativity, or emotional state?

By observing your unique response to the moon, you begin to build a foundation of self-awareness that will inform how you personalize your lunar journey.

Aligning the Lunar Phases with Your Personal Goals

One of the most empowering ways to personalize your lunar journey is by aligning the moon's phases with your personal goals and intentions. Each lunar phase offers a different type of energy that can support specific actions, mindsets, and healing practices.

New Moon: Setting Personal Intentions

The New Moon is a powerful time for setting intentions and beginning new projects. But rather than relying on generic goals, this phase is an opportunity to get deeply personal with your intentions. What do you truly want to cultivate in your life? Whether it's spiritual growth, healing relationships, or developing self-confidence, use the New Moon as a time to plant the seeds of your personal desires.

How to Personalize Your New Moon Ritual:

- Write down goals that speak to your heart, not just to external achievements. What inner growth do you want to cultivate? What emotional or spiritual transformations are you seeking?
- Create a New Moon ritual that feels authentic to you. This could involve journaling, lighting a candle, or even creating vision boards with imagery that resonates with your goals.
- Incorporate a personal symbol or item into your ritual—such as a crystal, photo, or heirloom—that holds special meaning to you and can anchor your intention-setting process.

Waxing Moon: Building Momentum for Your Unique Path

As the moon grows in light, you'll feel a natural pull toward action and growth. However, it's important to build momentum in a way that aligns with your personal pace and priorities. While some people thrive on taking big, bold steps during the Waxing Moon, others might need to focus on more subtle, internal progress.

How to Personalize Your Waxing Moon Practice:

- Reflect on your personal approach to growth. Do you prefer steady, incremental progress, or are you energized by bold action? Honor your personal rhythm during this phase.
- Choose rituals that support your growth in a way that feels nourishing. For example, you might feel drawn to energizing breathwork, a morning walk, or a self-reflective journal practice that keeps you focused without overwhelming you.
- Set small, actionable goals that feel aligned with your personal journey, rather than trying to match someone else's pace. Progress is deeply personal and should be celebrated at every step, no matter how big or small.

Full Moon: Reflecting on Personal Success and Releasing What No Longer Fits

The Full Moon brings an opportunity for reflection and release. But to personalize this phase, it's important to reflect on what success and achievement mean to you. Your definition of success may not match societal norms, and that's okay. The Full Moon is a time to honor your personal accomplishments and recognize the inner growth you've achieved, even if it doesn't align with traditional markers of success.

How to Personalize Your Full Moon Practice:

- Celebrate personal milestones that hold meaning for you—whether they are related to emotional healing, creative breakthroughs, or simply getting through a challenging period.

- Engage in a release ritual that is deeply personal. This might involve writing a letter to yourself, listing limiting beliefs or habits, and then symbolically releasing them through burning, tearing, or burying.
- Reflect on what no longer fits in your life, whether it's an outdated mindset, an old goal, or a relationship dynamic. Focus on releasing what feels misaligned, making space for new energy in the coming cycle.

Waning Moon: Embracing Rest and Deep Self-Care

As the moon wanes, it invites you to slow down and release excess energy. This phase is about deep self-care and introspection, but the way you choose to rest and restore should be tailored to your personal needs.

How to Personalize Your Waning Moon Practice:

- Reflect on what type of rest is most nourishing to you. Do you crave physical rest through sleep and relaxation, or do you find mental and emotional rest through meditation, reading, or creativity?
- Create a nighttime ritual that feels restorative. This could include a calming herbal tea, a candlelit bath, or a short meditation that helps you release the day's stress.
- Incorporate grounding practices that make you feel centered. If physical grounding feels right, spend time outdoors or practice yoga. If emotional grounding resonates, journaling or connecting with loved ones may feel more supportive.

Intuitive Ritual Creation: Listening to Your Inner Guidance

One of the most powerful ways to personalize your lunar journey is by trusting your intuition when it comes to creating rituals and practices. While this book offers a variety of rituals aligned with each lunar phase, your inner wisdom knows what will serve you best in the moment.

Steps to Intuitive Ritual Creation:

1. Tune In: Before creating a ritual, take a few moments to center yourself. Close your eyes, take a few deep breaths, and ask yourself what you need at this moment. Is it rest? Focus? Healing? Clarity? Allow your intuition to guide you.
2. Choose Elements That Speak to You: Based on your intuitive sense, choose elements for your ritual that feel aligned. This could be herbs, candles, crystals, or even music. Trust your instincts when selecting these elements, even if they differ from traditional suggestions.
3. Simplify or Elaborate as Needed: Your ritual doesn't need to follow a strict format. If you're feeling tired, a simple candle-lighting ritual with a single intention might be enough. If you're seeking deep healing, you might feel drawn to a longer, more elaborate practice. Let your intuition shape the structure of your ritual.

Journaling Your Lunar Journey: A Tool for Personal Growth

Journaling is a powerful tool for reflecting on your lunar journey and tracking your personal growth. By regularly documenting your thoughts, emotions, and experiences, you can gain insights into how the lunar cycles influence your life and identify patterns in your energy, moods, and desires.

Journaling Prompts for Your Lunar Journey:

- New Moon: What intentions do I want to set for this cycle? What new beginnings am I ready to embrace?
- Waxing Moon: What steps can I take to nurture my intentions? How can I support my personal growth during this phase?
- Full Moon: What am I most proud of during this cycle? What have I accomplished or learned?
- Waning Moon: What am I ready to release? How can I honor the need for rest and renewal?

Use these prompts to create a dedicated lunar journal, where you can track your thoughts, feelings, and personal insights. Over time, you'll develop a deeper understanding of your lunar journey and how it supports your growth and healing.

Incorporating Astrology and Numerology into Your Lunar Journey

For those who feel drawn to astrology or numerology, these practices can offer additional layers of personalization to your lunar journey. By exploring your astrological birth chart or working with your life path number, you can gain deeper insights into how the lunar phases align with your unique energetic blueprint.

Astrology and the Lunar Phases:

- New Moon in Your Sun Sign: Pay attention to when the New Moon falls in your sun sign, as this marks a powerful time for personal transformation and setting intentions aligned with your true self.
- Full Moon in Your Rising Sign: The Full Moon in your rising sign can offer deep emotional insights and highlight areas of personal growth. Reflect on how this energy influences your self-perception and relationships.

Numerology and the Lunar Cycles:

- Personal Year Number: If you work with numerology, consider how your current personal year number influences your lunar journey. For example, a personal year of "1" aligns with new beginnings and growth, making New Moon rituals especially potent.
- Life Path Number: Your life path number can offer insights into your overall approach to the lunar cycles. A life path number of "4," for example, might be drawn to rituals focused on stability and grounding, while a life path "7" may seek spiritual reflection and deeper meaning during the lunar phases.

Final Thoughts: Trusting Your Unique Lunar Path

As you continue your journey with the moon, remember that your experience is entirely unique. The moon offers us a mirror to reflect on our inner world,

18

Finding Balance in the Cycles - A Path to Healing and Wellness

As we've journeyed through the phases of the moon and explored how each phase influences not only our external world but also our inner landscape, we see that everything in life moves in cycles. Whether it's the changing tides, shifting seasons, or the ebb and flow of our emotions and energy, we are part of a larger, interconnected rhythm.

In this concluding chapter, I invite you to reflect on the journey we've taken together—exploring the natural phases of the moon, harnessing the energy of herbs, and incorporating spiritual practices that align with these cycles. It becomes clear that wellness is not about achieving perfection or maintaining a constant state of bliss. Instead, it's about embracing the natural cycles of change, healing, growth, and release that are inherent to our human experience.

Honoring the Cycles of Life and Nature

Throughout this book, we've observed how the moon mirrors the cycles of life. Just as the moon's phases offer unique opportunities for reflection, healing, and transformation, so too do our personal cycles. These phases are more than celestial changes in the night sky; they reflect the broader patterns that shape our lives—beginnings, growth, culmination, and release.

One of the most important lessons I've learned through my own journey is that we are not meant to be in a constant state of productivity or brightness. There are moments when we feel energized and ready to conquer our goals, and other times when we must slow down, rest, and reflect. Both states are equally valuable and necessary in our healing process.

When we honor these cycles instead of resisting them, we find ourselves in a state of flow, moving with life's natural rhythms. This is where true healing begins—not in striving for constant progress, but in accepting that wellness is a journey, not a destination. By aligning ourselves with the cycles of nature, we can cultivate more balance and ease in our lives.

Grounding Yourself in the Present Moment

One of the greatest teachings of the moon is the importance of being present. Just as the moon remains steady in its orbit—moving through phases of light and shadow—we too can find grounding in the present moment, regardless of where we are on our path.

In today's fast-paced world, we are often pushed to achieve more, be more, and do more. But holistic wellness teaches us to slow down, listen to our bodies, and ground ourselves in the here and now. When we connect with the cycles of the moon, we are reminded to pause, breathe, and align with the natural rhythms of life.

Grounding practices—such as meditation, breathwork, or simply spending time in nature—are essential tools for restoring balance and clarity. These practices help us stay centered, even in the face of life's challenges, and guide us back to a place of peace and inner calm. The moon's cycles encourage us to practice mindfulness, be gentle with ourselves, and trust that each phase, whether light or dark, has a purpose in our journey.

The Power of Intention and Self-Compassion

A recurring theme throughout this journey has been the power of intention. Whether it's setting goals during the New Moon or releasing burdens under the Full Moon, intention is the driving force that connects us to our deeper desires and guides our actions.

Intentions are not rigid goals. They are the seeds of possibility, planted in the fertile soil of our awareness, allowing them to grow in their own time. Just as the moon moves at its own pace, so too does our healing. By setting clear intentions, we create a framework for growth while practicing self-compassion when things don't unfold as we expected.

Self-compassion is a vital part of this process. It allows us to embrace both our successes and our setbacks with kindness, understanding that healing is not a linear path. Like the moon, we will wax and wane, experiencing cycles of high energy, growth, and periods of rest. In these moments of ebb and flow, it's important to treat ourselves with the same care and compassion that we extend to others.

Healing is a deeply personal journey, and just as each phase of the moon offers different lessons, so too does each phase of our lives.

Integrating Holistic Practices and Rituals

In this book, we have explored holistic practices such as herbal remedies, meditation, breathwork, and more—tools that align with the phases of the moon to create a foundation for holistic wellness. These practices are meant to be integrated into your life in a way that feels authentic and supportive to your personal journey.

The key to lasting healing lies in consistency and adaptability. The moon's phases offer us a natural rhythm to align with, but it's important to remember that wellness is not one-size-fits-all. Your needs will change with the cycles, and what resonates with you during one phase may not during another.

As you move forward, I encourage you to take the practices and rituals that resonate with you and make them your own. Whether it's creating a New Moon intention-setting ceremony, drinking herbal teas during the Full Moon, or practicing breathwork for release during the Waning Moon, these tools are here to support you in your ongoing wellness journey.

Personal Reflection: My Own Healing Journey

In my own life, the moon has been a constant guide, especially during the most difficult times. In moments of darkness, when uncertainty and fear felt overwhelming, the moon reminded me that just as it moves through phases of shadow and light, so too would I. The moon taught me that healing is cyclical—that growth happens even in the quiet, unseen moments of rest and reflection.

There have been times when I felt strong, capable, and full of light, and there have been moments when I felt lost in the darkness. But through it all, the moon showed me that each phase is necessary and that I was always moving forward, even when it didn't feel like it.

The rituals and practices I've shared throughout this book have been instrumental in my healing journey. They have grounded me, provided clarity when I needed it, and offered a sense of peace and comfort. It is my deepest hope that these practices will offer you the same. In your moments of darkness, I hope you find solace in knowing that, like the moon, your light will return.

Bringing It All Together: Healing Through Holistic Alignment

As we close this chapter and this book, I invite you to reflect on your own relationship with the moon and with yourself. What have you discovered about your personal cycles? How can you honor the natural rhythms of your body, mind, and spirit as you move forward?

Healing is not about erasing our struggles or striving for perfection. It's about embracing the wholeness of who we are—the light and the shadow, the joy and the sorrow. The moon reminds us that there is beauty in every phase, and that we are not defined by any single moment, but by the entirety of our journey.

As you continue your path, may the practices and rituals we've explored together offer you grounding, clarity, and inspiration. Remember, healing takes time, and just like the moon, you are always evolving. Trust the process, be kind to yourself, and honor the cycles within and around you.

Final Thoughts: The Journey Ahead

The journey doesn't end here. The wisdom, tools, and insights shared in this book are meant to be lifelong companions on your path to holistic wellness. The moon will continue to rise and set, offering you endless opportunities for reflection, growth, and healing.

Remember to trust in the natural rhythms of life. Healing takes time, but with each new lunar cycle, you have the opportunity to deepen your connection to yourself and the world around you. Be patient, honor your journey, and know that with each phase, you are stepping more fully into your power and wholeness.

Thank you for joining me on this journey. May the cycles of the moon continue to illuminate your path and offer you peace, balance, and healing in every phase of your life.

Epilogue

A Word from the Author

I'm Samantha Peterein, and if you've found your way to this book, I believe there is a reason. There's something about the moon, nature, and the ebb and flow of life that speaks to us on a soul-deep level, isn't there? I've felt that connection for as long as I can remember, but it wasn't until I faced some of my life's most difficult challenges that I truly leaned into it.

My journey has not been without its struggles. Like many, I've dealt with anxiety, depression, and a health diagnosis that turned my world upside down. I was the one who tried to keep it all together for everyone else, but inside, I was unraveling. In those moments of feeling lost and overwhelmed, I found myself searching for something—anything—that could ground me and help me navigate the chaos. That's when I turned to the moon, to nature, and to the ancient wisdom of herbs for guidance.

The moon's quiet, predictable cycles became a mirror for my own emotional ups and downs, showing me that just like its phases, life moves through cycles of growth, release, and renewal. The more I aligned with the moon's energy and the healing power of herbs, the more I found peace, clarity, and a deeper sense of purpose. The moon reminded me that it's okay to ebb and flow, to rise and retreat, and that each phase has its own unique beauty and wisdom.

This book is the result of my journey—an offering from my heart to yours. It's a collection of practices, rituals, and insights that have helped me find balance and healing. My hope is that it inspires you to pause, reflect, and reconnect with the natural rhythms that surround you. Whether you're seeking healing, clarity, or a deeper connection to the universe, I believe the moon and nature have gifts to offer you, just as they have for me.

This is your invitation to embrace the cycles of life, to honor where you are, and to trust that growth and healing are always within reach. You don't need to have it all figured out. The beauty of these practices is that they meet you where you are, whether you're in a phase of planting new seeds, nurturing growth, or letting go of what no longer serves you.

Thank you for allowing me to share this journey with you. I hope you find as much beauty, comfort, and wisdom in these pages as I've found in my own path to healing. May the moon's light and nature's embrace guide you, and may you always feel grounded in your own cycles of growth and renewal.

With love and gratitude,
  Samantha Peterein

Glossary of Key Terms

Lunar Phases

- New Moon: The first phase of the moon when it is not visible from Earth. Represents new beginnings, intention-setting, and potential. A time for planting seeds for future growth.
- Waxing Crescent: The phase following the New Moon, during which the moon's light begins to grow. Symbolizes growth, action, and building momentum toward goals.
- First Quarter: The phase halfway between the New Moon and Full Moon. A time of challenges, decisions, and progress, requiring commitment to your goals.
- Waxing Gibbous: The moon is nearly full and light continues to increase. This phase represents refinement, adjustment, and preparation for culmination.
- Full Moon: The peak of lunar energy, when the moon is fully illuminated. Associated with culmination, reflection, release, and celebrating achievements.
- Waning Gibbous: The phase following the Full Moon, where the light starts to decrease. This is a time for introspection, processing emotions, and letting go of what no longer serves you.
- Last Quarter: The phase halfway between the Full Moon and New Moon. It represents deep release, emotional healing, and removing obstacles to prepare for a new cycle.
- Waning Crescent: The final phase before the New Moon. A time for rest, surrender, and preparation for the new cycle to begin. Often associated

with endings and closure.

Herbs and Plants

- Ashwagandha (Withania somnifera): A powerful adaptogen used to reduce stress, improve energy, and support mental clarity. Often incorporated into tonics for overall wellness.
- Basil (Ocimum basilicum): A fragrant herb used for purification, protection, and mental clarity. Commonly added to teas or baths for its uplifting energy.
- Burdock Root (Arctium lappa): A detoxifying herb used to cleanse the blood and support skin health. Often included in tonics for liver support and purification.
- Chamomile (Matricaria chamomilla): A calming herb known for its gentle sedative properties. Used to reduce anxiety, support sleep, and soothe the digestive system.
- Cinnamon (Cinnamomum spp.): A warming spice used for prosperity, protection, and circulation. Often used in rituals and teas for attracting abundance and stimulating the senses.
- Dandelion (Taraxacum officinale): A nourishing herb for detoxification and liver health. Its leaves and roots are used in teas and tinctures for grounding and release.
- Frankincense (Boswellia spp.): A sacred resin used for protection, meditation, and spiritual connection. Burned as incense or added to oil blends for purification and healing.
- Ginger (Zingiber officinale): A warming herb for digestion, circulation, and energy. Often used in teas for energizing the body and clearing stagnant energy.
- Ginseng (Panax spp.): A powerful adaptogen used to increase energy, stamina, and mental clarity. Frequently added to tonics and teas for vitality.

- Gotu Kola (Centella asiatica): A rejuvenating herb used to support brain function, mental clarity, and skin health. Frequently added to teas for its anti-aging properties.
- Juniper (Juniperus spp.): A protective herb used for cleansing and warding off negative energy. Burned as incense or used in smudge sticks for purification.
- Jasmine (Jasminum spp.): A sweet, fragrant flower associated with love, sensuality, and relaxation. Commonly used in teas and oils for calming and uplifting the spirit.
- Lavender (Lavandula spp.): A calming herb used for relaxation, sleep, and emotional balance. Frequently added to baths, teas, and oils for peace and serenity.
- Lemon Balm (Melissa officinalis): A soothing herb used for anxiety, stress relief, and emotional balance. Added to teas or tinctures for calming the mind and heart.
- Lemongrass (Cymbopogon citratus): A refreshing herb used for purification, cleansing, and clarity. Often used in teas or diffused for its energizing and clearing properties.
- Mint (Mentha spp.): A refreshing herb used for mental clarity, digestion, and energy clearing. Commonly added to teas or baths for cleansing and revitalization.
- Mugwort (Artemisia vulgaris): A powerful herb used for intuition, dream work, and spiritual insight. Often burned as incense or added to teas and tinctures for reflection and mental clarity.
- Nettle (Urtica dioica): A nutrient-rich herb used for detoxification, energy, and circulation. Often added to teas or tonics for strengthening and revitalizing the body.
- Passion Flower (Passiflora incarnata): A calming herb used to soothe anxiety, promote sleep, and enhance emotional balance. Frequently included in teas and tinctures for relaxation.
- Peppermint (Mentha piperita): A refreshing herb used for clarity, digestion, and respiratory support. Added to teas or inhaled for mental focus and clearing congestion.

- Rose (Rosa spp.): A fragrant flower used for love, beauty, and emotional healing. Often used in teas, baths, and oils for heart-centered rituals and relaxation.
- Rosemary (Rosmarinus officinalis): A protective and invigorating herb used for memory, focus, and purification. Frequently added to teas, baths, or burned as incense for cleansing and focus.
- Sage (Salvia spp.): Includes multiple varieties like white, blue, and black sage. Used for purification, protection, and spiritual connection. Often burned in smudge sticks for cleansing and clearing negative energy.
- Skullcap (Scutellaria lateriflora): A calming herb used to ease stress, anxiety, and tension. Often added to teas and tinctures for relaxation and mental clarity.
- Valerian (Valeriana officinalis): A strong sedative herb used to promote deep sleep and relaxation. Commonly included in teas and tinctures for calming the nervous system.

Magick and Rituals

- Affirmation: A positive statement or declaration made with intention, used to align energy and manifest desired outcomes.
- Manifestation: The process of turning thoughts, desires, or intentions into reality through focused energy, action, and intention.
- Ritual: A series of intentional actions, often performed with symbolic meaning, to create a connection with spiritual or energetic forces. Rituals are often used to mark phases of the moon or support manifestation.
- Grounding: A practice that involves connecting your energy to the Earth to promote stability, calm, and centeredness. Grounding is often performed through meditation, visualization, or physical contact with nature.
- Intention: A focused desire or goal that guides thoughts, actions, and energy. Setting an intention is often the first step in manifestation or ritual practice.

- Energy Healing: A practice aimed at balancing or restoring the body's energy systems to promote physical, emotional, or spiritual well-being. Includes practices like Reiki, crystal healing, and sound therapy.
- Smudging: A ritual practice of burning herbs (such as sage, rosemary, or cedar) to purify a space, object, or person. Often used for energy clearing and protection.

Additional Terms

- Lunar Journey: The personal path one takes in aligning with the moon's phases to enhance spiritual, emotional, and mental well-being. This can include rituals, meditations, and personalized practices.
- Empowerment Cycles: Phases or cycles of growth, reflection, and action that focus on personal empowerment, often aligning with lunar or life phases to enhance self-awareness and confidence.
- Customization of Rituals: The process of adapting traditional or personal rituals to fit unique intentions, goals, or spiritual practices. This could involve selecting herbs, setting specific intentions, or modifying meditations to align with one's personal journey.
- Life Phases & Lunar Practices: The concept of adapting lunar practices and rituals based on different stages of life, including changes in personal circumstances, goals, and emotional needs.

Recommended Resources for Further Exploration

As you continue your journey into the world of holistic wellness, lunar cycles, and herbal practices, there are many more incredible resources that can guide and support your growth. Whether you are looking to deepen your knowledge of herbalism, explore Ayurvedic teachings, or expand your understanding of traditional healing practices, the following books, teachers, and guides will offer valuable insights.

Books by the Author:

The Modern Herbalist's Guide: 30 Days to Healing and Harmony by Samantha Peterein

- This guide provides a practical and structured 30-day approach to integrating herbal remedies into your daily life. It's perfect for both beginners and those looking to deepen their connection to herbs and holistic healing.

Rooted in Healing: An Introduction to Herbs and Rituals for Wellness by Samantha Peterein

- This introduction serves as a gentle guide for anyone wanting to explore the basics of herbalism and spiritual rituals. It focuses on accessible herbal remedies, rituals for self-care, and ways to connect more deeply with nature and your own wellness journey.

Recommended Authors and Teachers:

Barbara O'Neil – General Herbalism

- Barbara O'Neil is an exceptional herbalist and natural health educator whose teachings blend science and tradition. Her books and lectures focus on the body's ability to heal itself using natural remedies, nutrition, and herbal practices. Her approach is accessible for those new to herbalism but also provides depth for seasoned practitioners.

Sahara Rose – Ayurveda and Modern Wellness

- Sahara Rose is a contemporary voice in Ayurvedic teachings, making this ancient practice accessible for modern audiences. Her work emphasizes understanding your Dosha (mind–body constitution) and integrating Ayurvedic principles into daily life. Sahara's books and podcasts are excellent resources for anyone looking to deepen their knowledge of Ayurveda and personal wellness.

Additional Books and Authors:

"The Complete Herbal Tutor" by Anne McIntyre

- A comprehensive resource on Western herbalism, this book offers an in-depth look at various herbs and their medicinal properties. It also provides practical advice for growing, harvesting, and preparing herbs in different ways.

"Medical Herbalism: The Science and Practice of Herbal Medicine" by David Hoffmann

- A respected authority in the field of herbal medicine, David Hoffmann provides a bridge between traditional herbal knowledge and modern scientific research. This book is ideal for those looking to understand the therapeutic actions of herbs on a deeper level.

"Eat Feel Fresh: A Contemporary, Plant-Based Ayurvedic Cookbook" by Sahara Rose

- This book offers a refreshing take on Ayurveda with an emphasis on plant-based eating. It's a great resource for anyone looking to integrate Ayurvedic nutrition into their daily routine while learning about how food and herbs can balance the Doshas.

"The Moon Book: Lunar Magic to Change Your Life" by Sarah Faith Gottesdiener

- A guide to aligning your spiritual practice with lunar cycles, including rituals, spells, and journal prompts.

"The Complete Guide to Self-Care" by Kiki Ely

- A holistic approach to wellness, focusing on self-care routines, including baths, herbal remedies, and energy healing.

Resources for Traditional Chinese Medicine (TCM):

"The Web That Has No Weaver: Understanding Chinese Medicine" by Ted J. Kaptchuk

- This classic book introduces the core concepts of TCM, including Yin and Yang, the Five Elements, and Qi (life force energy). It's perfect for those interested in understanding how TCM integrates with holistic practices like acupuncture and herbal medicine.

"Healing with Whole Foods: Asian Traditions and Modern Nutrition" by Paul Pitchford

- This book merges traditional Chinese dietary principles with modern nutritional science, offering a holistic approach to healing through food. It's a great resource for anyone looking to integrate TCM with daily eating habits.

Online Platforms and Courses:

- Herbal Academy – Offers a variety of online courses, from beginner to advanced levels, focusing on herbalism, botany, and holistic health practices.
- Sahara Rose's Dosha Quiz – Found on her website, this free quiz helps you discover your Ayurvedic Dosha and learn how to balance your mind and body according to ancient Ayurvedic wisdom.
- Mountain Rose Herbs – A trusted online store for sourcing high-quality herbs, essential oils, and herbal crafting supplies. Their blog also offers recipes and guides for incorporating herbal remedies into your wellness

routine.

By engaging with these resources, you can continue your exploration of herbalism, Ayurveda, Traditional Chinese Medicine, and holistic wellness in ways that align with both ancient traditions and modern needs. Each book and guide offers unique insights that complement your personal practice, deepening your understanding of how nature's wisdom can support your health and healing.